SLEEP

Problems and Solutions

SLEEP

Problems and Solutions

Quentin Regestein, M.D., David Ritchie,
and the Editors of
Consumer Reports Books

Consumers Union
Mount Vernon, New York

The ideas, procedures, and suggestions contained in this book are not intended to replace the services of a physician. All matters regarding your health require medical supervision, and you should consult a physician before adopting the procedures in this book. Any application of the treatments set forth herein are at the reader's discretion, and neither the authors nor the publisher assume any responsibility or liability therefor.

The cases and examples cited in this book are based on actual situations and real people. Names and identifying details have been changed to protect privacy.

Library of Congress Cataloging-in-Publication Data
Regestein, Quentin R.
Sleep: problems and solutions / Quentin Regestein, David Ritchie,
and the editors of Consumer Reports Books.
p. cm.
Includes index.
ISBN 0-89043-065-9. — ISBN 0-89043-055-1 (pbk.)
1. Sleep disorders—Popular works. I. Ritchie, David, 1952 Sept.
18- II. Consumer Reports Books. III. Title.
RC547.R44 1989
616.8'49—dc 19   89-30861
                                                                CIP

Design by Jeffrey L. Ward

Manufactured in the United States of America

Figure 3 on p. 42 reprinted by permission: Juergen Aschoff, "Desynchronization and Resynchronization of Human Circadian Rhythms," *Aerospace Medicine* 40:8, August 1969; copyright © 1969, *Aerospace Medicine*. All rights reserved.

Figure 10 on p. 139 reprinted by permission: Nathaniel Kleitman, *Sleep and Wakefulness*, The University of Chicago Press, Chicago; copyright © 1939, 1963 The University of Chicago Press. All rights reserved.

Figure 11 on p. 198 reprinted by permission: Anthony Cales, et al., "Chronic Hypnotic Drug Use," *Journal of the American Medical Association* 227:5, February 4, 1974, pp. 513–17; copyright © 1974, American Medical Association. All rights reserved.

Sleep: Problems and Solutions is a Consumer Reports Book published by Consumers Union, the nonprofit organization that publishes *Consumer Reports,* the monthly magazine of test reports, product Ratings, and buying guidance. Established in 1936, Consumers Union is chartered under the Not-For-Profit Corporation Law of the State of New York.

The purposes of Consumers Union, as stated in its charter, are to provide consumers with information and counsel on consumer goods and services, to give information on all matters relating to the expenditure of the family income, and to initiate and to cooperate with individual and group efforts seeking to create and maintain decent living standards.

Consumers Union derives its income solely from the sale of *Consumer Reports* and other publications. In addition, expenses of occasional public service efforts may be met, in part, by nonrestrictive, noncommercial contributions, grants, and fees. Consumers Union accepts no advertising or product samples and is not beholden in any way to any commercial interest. Its Ratings and reports are solely for the use of the readers of its publications. Neither the Ratings nor the reports nor any Consumers Union publications, including this book, may be used in advertising or for any commercial purpose. Consumers Union will take all steps open to it to prevent such uses of its materials, its name, or the name of *Consumer Reports.*

BOMC offers recordings and compact discs, cassettes
and records. For information and catalog write to
BOMR, Camp Hill, PA 17012.

Contents

Introduction

Good health requires good sleep. Sound sleep restores the body and mind; poor sleep leaves the body fatigued and the mind dull. Yet people who regularly sleep well take their nightly rest for granted. For them, "sleep that knits up the raveled sleave of care," as Shakespeare wrote, comes easily and naturally. But as many as one out of seven adults suffers from poor-quality sleep. For them, lack of sleep impairs not only physical health, but also family life, emotional well-being, and job and career.

In 1986 a panel of sleep specialists from the American Sleep Disorders Association estimated that, based on the patients they treated and their personal observations, about 30 million Americans suffer from insomnia. The panel's judgments, as well as telephone and other surveys, indicate that sleeplessness and sleep-related problems are everywhere in our society. Unfortunately, many people who suffer from poor-quality sleep either never realize that their constant fatigue is caused by a sleep problem or assume that nothing can be done. Once recognized, however, most sleep problems can be remedied.

Sleep Problems and Solutions is a guide not only to understanding sleep and sleep disturbances and disorders, but also to learning what treatments are available for some of these problems.

The most common problems, such as insomnia, are discussed, as well as some less-usual but significant disorders. If you are dissatisfied with your energy level during the day or the quality of your sleep at night, or if the well-being of a family member or friend concerns you, *Sleep Problems and Solutions* can help you understand the causes of poor sleep and give you guidelines on what can be done to treat them.

Over the past twenty-five years, research has revealed a great deal about basic sleep processes such as sleep phases, dreaming or rapid eye movement (REM) sleep, and the biochemistry of sleep. What scientists at one time considered to be a simple slowing down of the brain and body is now known to be a complex orchestration of neurochemicals, hormones, biological clocks, and various body chemicals and systems. Knowledge of those mechanisms can help you understand what goes wrong during disturbed sleep.

After studying the fundamentals of sleep, researchers were able to define numerous sleep disorders, then clinicians were able to establish a range of treatments for most of them. Yet effective treatment for sleep problems still involves intangibles, including how well the physician and patient work together and how well treatment is individualized. *Sleep Problems and Solutions* provides you with information that helps you approach your treatment knowledgeably.

Insomnia, the most common sleep complaint, is a symptom with hundreds of causes, including everything from street noise to frequent urination to physical illness. Irregularities in biological clocks create poor sleep much more frequently than people generally recognize, and the side effects of everyday drugs can play a role as well. Mental disorders can profoundly disrupt sleep. Insomnia, in fact, is one diagnostic clue to depression. Hormonal disturbances and menopause can also bring about or aggravate sleeplessness. Therefore, identifying the exact cause or causes of insomnia sometimes requires persistence. Treatment itself is usually highly individualized, although a sleep hygiene program is generally regarded as a good starting place for everyone with insomnia.

Sleep hygiene includes such relatively simple measures as

keeping a chart of when you sleep, eliminating drugs that affect sleep (caffeine, alcohol, and nicotine, for example), establishing a regular exercise program, and setting a regular sleep schedule. These self-help measures alone can greatly increase your chances of sleeping well regularly.

Still, you must take care to determine what causes poor-quality sleep. Chronic fatigue or sleepiness may not be caused simply by lack of sleep but may be symptoms of an unrecognized, underlying disorder. For example, sleepiness and sudden episodes of deep sleep characterize *narcolepsy,* a well-defined disorder that often requires medication. In addition, the physician and narcoleptic must regularly adjust the treatment to accommodate irregular schedules, additional responsibilities, and other changes in daily life.

Sleep apnea is another serious and potentially dangerous cause of sleepiness that usually goes unrecognized by the person who has it. The breathing of sleep apnea victims stops frequently and intermittently during sleep—sometimes hundreds of times a night and occasionally for one full minute or longer. Sleep apnea sufferers feel tired and lethargic. Among many other characteristics, they snore very loudly; often their partners bring them in for treatment. If sleep apnea is suspected, professional diagnosis and treatment should be sought as soon as possible.

Many chronic fatigue or sleep problems, including jet lag, arise from the disruption of *circadian rhythms,* which are regulated by the biological clocks. These 24-hour cycles of body temperature fluctuations, hormone secretions, enzyme activity, and other physiological functions govern patterns for sleep and wakefulness. Sound sleep depends on the internal timing and synchronization of these rhythms and on external cues that keep the "sleep clock" set (see chap. 3). When the cycles receive conflicting signals or become mistimed and out of phase, or when you shift your sleep-wake schedule suddenly and drastically, sleep problems and fatigue will result. Certain techniques can help you reset your "sleep clock" when its timekeeping is off, and there are even ways to minimize the chances that you will suffer from jet lag.

People generally take coffee and alcoholic beverages for

granted. However, caffeine or alcohol can severely disrupt the sleep of people who are sensitive to these substances, as can the nicotine in tobacco and some chemicals in over-the-counter and prescription medicines. As just mentioned, a basic prescription for better sleep involves eliminating caffeine and alcohol from the diet, quitting smoking, and stopping, gradually diminishing, or changing medications. Of course, you should *not* discontinue or alter a prescription medication on your own: You and your doctor can either change medications or devise a schedule for taking a sleep-disrupting prescription drug, adjusting its dosage to achieve better sleep. Giving up addictive habits, particularly drugs such as caffeine or nicotine, which cause withdrawal symptoms is never easy. This book provides some guidance for those trying to quit.

For some people, insomnia may well be connected to personality. Those who are overly sensitive to everyday stimuli may suffer from *hyperarousal insomnia,* which makes it harder to fall asleep or stay asleep. Despite persistent fatigue, the person may become resigned to insomnia as a way of life. But simple techniques such as regular exercise, progressive relaxation exercises, or even a hot bath before bed can lower the individual's arousal level and often bring relief. Such techniques involve no fundamental transformation of the personality; they require only some sustained effort to incorporate a few new routines into your daily schedule. This book includes a self-assessment test for hyperarousal insomnia and presents a program to help you cope with it, if necessary.

Older people frequently complain about daytime fatigue and poor-quality sleep, too. Insomnia generally increases as one ages, but the aging process should not condemn a person to chronic sleeplessness. Unfortunately, many older people habitually use sleeping pills to alleviate insomnia. Frequent reliance on sleeping pills may actually harm sleep quality. This book suggests techniques to help an older person achieve optimal and satisfying sleep without drugs.

Childhood-onset insomnia sufferers tend to have severe insomnia, although the specifics of each case vary widely. Causes often lie in some fundamental, organic anomaly of brain structure or body chemistry. The exact reasons for childhood-onset insomnia usually remain an enigma, which makes treatment difficult. Nevertheless, even if doctors cannot determine the exact cause, treatment is possible.

If "sleep charting" and other sleep hygiene techniques prove ineffective, or if you suspect a serious problem, you may need professional help. This book contains a short questionnaire designed to help you determine whether you should consult a sleep clinic for help. Although professional help does not usually involve psychotherapy, it can help when long-term emotional problems disrupt sleep or when all attempts to change sleep-disrupting habits have proven unsuccessful.

If you feel that you lack sufficient daily energy, if you think you sleep too much or not as well as you should, or if the restless slumber of a loved one disturbs you, *Sleep Problems and Solutions* can be your guide to better sleep. It shows how most sleep problems can be successfully treated. No matter how intractable a problem may seem, it is worth investigating the causes and seeking some remedies; this book provides you with a good starting point.

1

....

Sleep and Its Significance

Although everyone needs sound, refreshing sleep, a person who has problems sleeping is not alone. One Gallup poll indicated that roughly 38 million Americans often have trouble falling asleep at night. Another survey conducted at random in Los Angeles revealed the following:

- 4 percent of respondents described themselves as "insomniacs"
- 15 percent reported frequent difficulty in falling asleep, even if they did not specifically refer to insomnia
- 16 percent said they awakened at night and had trouble falling asleep again
- 18 percent complained of not getting enough sleep
- 16 percent said they felt tired during the day because of insufficient sleep at night
- 32 percent reported some combination of the above sleep problems

Yet surveys such as these tell us only how many people confess sleep problems to surveyors. Large-scale, landmark surveys conducted in the 1970s by the National Institutes of Health (NIH) provide us with some information about how many people actually obtain medication to remedy sleep problems.

The NIH surveys were designed demographically using rigorous sampling methods. Subjects were interviewed in detail about their use of psychotropic drugs (drugs that act on the mind), including sleeping pills. The surveys revealed that some 17 percent of the population described themselves as "bothered greatly" by insomnia. That works out to roughly 40 million people. The surveys also provided some clues about how many people were merely complaining about sleeplessness and how many were trying to do something about it. An estimated 7 percent of the population was using medication to achieve better sleep, according to the surveys. (This estimate does not include the untold millions who try drinking themselves to sleep nightly.) Medication is not the only treatment for insomnia, but it is the most common treatment.

At the opposite extreme are sleep disorders that involve continual sleep or drowsiness night and day. Unlike the insomnia sufferer, who has great difficulty falling asleep, a person with *hypersomnia* cannot awaken fully. Although large-scale surveys have yet to be done on the incidence of this problem, sleep-disorder clinics commonly find that at least half of their patients have hypersomnia, so we know that it is not rare.

The economic impact of sleep disorders is hard to calculate. How many people go to sleep at the wheel while driving or doze off while on the job or simply don't work as well as they might because of sleep disorders? Some statistics on worker performance suggest that many night workers sleep on the job. Consider that there is a peak of truck-driving accidents around 4:00 A.M., when drivers are probably not very alert, and that train engineers, while being monitored for sleep with portable polygraphs, have actually been found to fall asleep while operating trains. Many day workers are probably sleepy as well; witness the dozing commuters riding trains to work each weekday morning, trying to grab a short nap to make up for the sound, refreshing sleep their bodies somehow missed the night before.

Many people simply accept their insomnia or drowsiness, not knowing that it can be treated and relieved. Sometimes obtaining relief is difficult, but often it is merely a matter of getting rid of habits that discourage sleep.

DIFFERENT SLEEP FOR DIFFERENT TYPES

Why does anyone sleep at all? Why can't we just stay awake? Some biologists suggest that sleep provides an opportunity to conduct self-repair and purge the body of metabolic waste built up during the day's activities. Yet the body is capable of repairing itself and disposing of wastes during waking hours, so sleep does not seem necessary for such routine maintenance.

Maybe sleep kept our distant ancestors out of harm's way during the night when they could not see as well as their night-roaming predators. (It seems likely that large cats and other carnivores preyed on early humans; hominid skulls discovered recently in Africa exhibit neat round holes that correspond exactly in size and spacing to the teeth of leopards.) Thus nocturnal sleep might have increased humans' chances of survival and become part of human physiology and behavior, as the night sleepers survived to have more night-sleeping children. But a universal behavior such as sleep seems basic to life. Sleep may have arisen out of circadian rhythms, the daily physiological cycles that promote survival by helping the body coordinate biochemical events and use energy economically (see chap. 3).

However sleep originated, it is common to all mammals; more primitive animals, who have simpler nervous systems, have regular rest periods as well. Each species adapts sleep to its own ecological niche. Certain sharks, for example, congregate in undersea caves for mass sleep-ins, whereas whales doze at the surface, their blowholes above water to allow them to breathe. Some breeds of cattle sleep standing up, because to lie down would disrupt their digestive systems.

Some species sleep a lot and others sleep a little. Sluggish tree-dwelling animals like sloths and opossums may spend 18 to 20 hours per day asleep. By contrast, ground-dwelling species subject to predation, such as deer and antelope, may sleep only

2 to 3 hours at a time. They are light sleepers, too, because more prolonged and deeper sleep would give their natural enemies, such as big cats and humans, more opportunity to slip up on them undetected.

Sleep begins in utero for humans, as revealed by ultrasound pictures of the eye movements of the unborn. A newborn child sleeps about 16 hours per day on the average, but the sleep is broken up into six to eight episodes distributed more or less evenly across the 24-hour period. The child's sleeping periods start to lengthen when it's around four weeks old. By about six months, most children experience unbroken sleep during the night, with additional naps in the morning and afternoon, although some babies take longer to "settle," or sleep through the night. Daytime nap periods gradually diminish. By age six, children generally are awake all day and sleep roughly 10 hours per night.

HOW THE BODY REGULATES SLEEP

Much research has been done on the specific processes of the body that produce sleep. Certain parts of the brain induce sleep and wakefulness. In the final decade of the nineteenth century, researchers conducting autopsies on patients who had died from encephalitis (a viral disease that inflames the brain cells and often causes the victim to sleep excessively) began to suspect that a deep midline area of the brain that controls our most vital functions was also involved in producing sleep. Later research enlarged this view.

Actually, there seems to be a connected series of structures in the deep midline areas and along other way stations that extend through the central axis of the brain, and these structures relay information about things that affect sleep. The system integrates the many influences on sleep, such as the body's schedules, external perceptions, and internal sensations, into a control system for sleep. Information about how such systems affect sleep has been discovered mainly through decades of animal experimentation. For instance, researchers would destroy specific brain structures of a lab animal and then note how the animal slept. A cut through the axis of the brain at one level prevented the animal from awakening, for example, showing that brain structures below the level of the cut were responsible for wakefulness. The destruction of specific groups of cells in the brain might cause animals to miss certain stages of sleep or change brain-wave patterns or behavioral patterns associated with a particular stage of sleep.

The *hypothalamus* is one of those midline structures that controls sleep. It also plays a role in governing other functions, such as thirst, appetite, sexual arousal, and bodily timing systems. The *superchiasmatic nucleus,* a small group of nerve cells in the hypothalamus, is located near the point where the optic nerves from each eye come together, and it seems to play a critical role as a "sleep timer," telling a person when to go to bed and when to wake up.

Conceptual models of sleep have undergone a profound reevaluation in the last half century. Researchers in the 1930s presumed that sleep was an essentially passive state resulting from decreased sensory input: people simply slept because they had nothing to respond to. Before long it became apparent that more was involved than a passive response to diminished sensation. It appears that two separate systems determine an individual's sleep/wake cycle: one system promotes sleep and the other, the arousal system, promotes wakefulness. There is a daily ebb and flow of wakefulness based on interplay between sleep and arousal. Furthermore, the arousal system has subdivisions: one for the kind of wakefulness that occurs regularly after the sun comes up, and another for wakefulness that occurs at unscheduled times in the middle of the night—for example, to answer an unexpected phone call or to respond to the cries of a sick child.

The body's biochemical regulation of sleep has been studied intensively in the last 30 years and, like any subject of research, is looking more complex all the time. Initially, sleep researchers became intrigued with the notion that certain *neurotransmitters,* substances that help transmit nerve impulses, might be involved in controlling sleep. (*Adrenaline* is a well-known neurotransmitter.)

Neurotransmitters are manufactured in the nervous system through biochemical changes in substances obtained from food. The digestive system breaks down *proteins* into *amino acids*. These are refined along their path from the intestine, where they are absorbed, through the liver, the blood, and the nervous system to the nerve cell. Each nerve cell then produces a particular type of neurotransmitter and stores it until it is ready to discharge, or "fire."

When the nerve cell fires, it discharges its particular type of neurotransmitter into the space between it and the next nerve cell. This discharge is released in about .001 second and causes an electrochemical reaction that makes the next nerve cell discharge and activate other nerve cells. Thus electrical signals are sent through specific paths in the nervous system. By administering drugs to increase or decrease a particular neurotransmitter's action, researchers can tell how neurotransmitters affect an individual. For example, the drug reserpine, used now mainly to treat high blood pressure, makes some people depressed, showing that the neurotransmitters it affects are those that help regulate mood. When drugs that do the opposite of reserpine are given, the person may become manic.

Since each person's nervous system is different, with a profile of nerve cells that is unique to that individual, the effect of drugs on that person cannot be precisely predicted. A drug that changes neurotransmitters in a predictable way can have unpredictable effects in certain people.

One neurotransmitter, *serotonin,* is particularly important in the biochemistry of sleep. It also plays a role in many other functions of the nervous system, including the regulation of our moods, our sensitivity to pain, and our appetite for food. In some animals, serotonin appears to accumulate during deep sleep. Another substance involved in sleep is *noradrenaline,* the principal neurotransmitter of the brain. Yet another is *acetylcholine,* which controls electrical activity not only in the brain but also in other areas, such as the heart, gut, and skin (for instance, in the regulation of glands that produce skin secretions).

The levels of these neurotransmitters in our body are influenced by our diet and by certain drugs, such as some medications taken for high blood pressure, nasal stuffiness, or peptic ulcers. Some constituents of food, such as *tryptophan, tyrosine,* and *choline,* can affect sleep because they contain substances that are metabolic building blocks for neurotransmitters.

Health-food stores often claim that taking these substances may help you sleep. In fact, tryptophan, commonly touted as a sleep aid, does make many people drowsy about half an hour after they take it (see chap. 10). How it works is not clearly known. Since tryptophan is the amino acid from which serotonin is made, and since serotonin blood levels increase when more tryptophan is ingested, it could cause more serotonin to be produced in the central nervous system. On the other hand, tryptophan could stimulate hormones in the intestine. These digestive hormones might as a side effect make you drowsy.

Recently, certain peptides have also been studied for their effects on sleep. A *peptide* is a short chain of amino acids. One sleep-making peptide is manufactured in the intestine by bacteria residing there, in much the same way that other intestinal bacteria produce vitamin K (a blood-clotting agent). This bacteria-made peptide induces deep sleep. Possibly other substances, secreted by the nervous system in ever-increasing amounts the longer one remains awake, also play a part in inducing sleep. One such substance is called *delta-sleep-inducing peptide,* or DSIP. DSIP is probably made in the nervous system and can make one sleep more deeply, thereby inducing greater wakefulness during the day.

SLEEP PATTERNS AND SLEEP STRUCTURES

Although the average duration of sleep for adults is roughly 7½ hours, the number of hours can vary considerably from one person to another. Some people require much less sleep than others. Napoleon is said to have functioned well on only 4 or

5 hours of sleep per night, whereas Albert Einstein required 10 hours or more.

Studies of twins suggest that the length of a person's nightly sleep is, in part, genetic. Whether a person is a long sleeper or a short sleeper remains, like a physiological fingerprint, largely constant throughout his or her life. Sleep hours may vary from night to night, but they average about the same from one month to another. Sleep specialists documented one case of a man who kept records of each hour he slept for two years, including naps. His average sleeping time per 24-hour period was the same for the second year as for the first, down to the second decimal place.

The *polygraph,* an instrument that measures electrical activity in the brain, can track the progress of sleep. Small electrodes are taped to the scalp of a sleeping person and around the eyes, under the chin, and elsewhere. Wires attached to the electrodes feed information to the polygraph on electrical activity taking place in the brain, eyes, and muscles. The instrument records the data in the form of ink trails on a moving roll of paper. The record from the scalp electrodes is called an *electroencephalogram,* or EEG. Brain-wave frequency (oscillations or cycles per second) and voltage (height) are shown on the EEG. The brain does not generate much electricity by industrial standards; its electrical output is measured in microvolts, or millionths of a volt. (An ordinary wall socket, by comparison, delivers 110 volts.) The polygraph is sensitive enough to pick up relatively faint signals and amplify them to make a readable record of brain activity.

Scalp electrodes pick up electrical activity from the billions of neurons that fire or discharge while the brain goes about its business during wakefulness and sleep. The brain must analyze information streaming in from the various sense organs and integrate it with data from deeper levels of the nervous system that govern memory, emotion, or instinct. The brain also suppresses inappropriate or antisocial reflexes that might otherwise happen automatically, such as urination or outbursts of anger. Simultaneously, it prepares and coordinates behavioral responses. The brain's basic task is to mediate between a person's inner requirements and the demands of the outside world. All this activity means that at any given moment a neuron may be engaged in a different task from its neighbor's.

Understandably, a scalp electrode monitoring this lively complexity during wakefulness is almost certain to register nothing but noise. The many tasks have organization, but together they are hard to keep track of—imagine trying to listen to several radios playing simultaneously!

This picture changes, however, as a person lies down, closes his or her eyes, and prepares to sleep. The cacophony of firing neurons diminishes. The nerve cells begin to fire more in rhythm. Alpha wave rhythms emerge from the neuronal noise and are picked up by the scalp electrodes.

The final record of a night's sleep on an EEG, condensed from the recordings of brain waves, eye movement, and muscle activity, is called a *somnogram* and looks much like a silhouette of a skyscraper-filled city landscape. The heights of the different "buildings" represent different stages of sleep (see fig. 1).

Now imagine you are hooked up to an EEG while preparing for a night's sleep. What might the machine record?

When you are fully awake, the EEG would show noisy irregularity within a narrow range of low voltage. This pattern means you are alert; eye-movement patterns would show that you are constantly using your eyes to monitor your surroundings.

As you close your eyes, the pattern changes. The needle on the EEG records definite cycles, about 8 to 12 per second, and the peaks on the graph move farther apart. Oscillations or "waves" on the graph grow wider, meaning that voltage has increased.

The rhythmical pattern of waves of 8 to 12 cycles per second is called the *alpha rhythm,* so named by Hans Berger, the psychiatrist who first described brain waves. Alpha waves are observed in the EEG when you are awake but calm—usually with your eyes closed, because focusing on visual images would require the brain to process visual information. This would bring about increased activity among the neurons, thus obscuring the observation of the underlying alpha waves. Alpha waves are

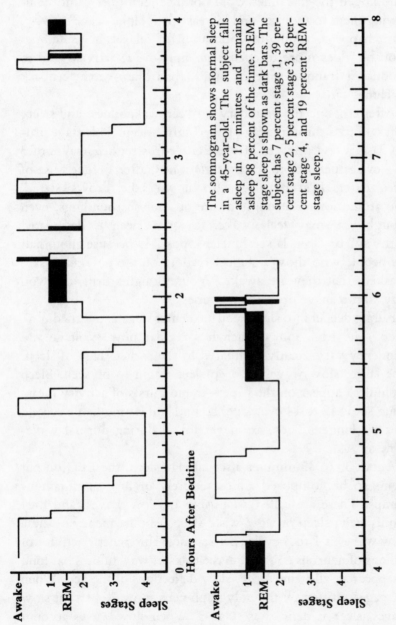

The somnogram shows normal sleep in a 45-year-old. The subject falls asleep in 17 minutes and remains asleep 88 percent of the time. REM-stage sleep is shown as dark bars. The subject has 7 percent stage 1, 39 percent stage 2, 5 percent stage 3, 18 percent stage 4, and 19 percent REM-stage sleep.

Figure 1 Somnogram of polygraph activity during a typical night's sleep.

the hallmark of calm wakefulness. Alpha rhythms enjoyed a fad some years ago, when feedback machines were sold to buyers who hoped the machines would bring them inner calm by allowing them to monitor and increase their alpha-wave activity. As it happens, assiduous application of relaxation techniques probably does more to encourage alpha-wave activity, and to produce a tranquil state of mind, than brain-wave feedback machines can.

After crossing the boundary between wakefulness and sleep, you will pass through stage 1, or "light" sleep. This stage usually lasts a few minutes. The EEG records regular waves of 3 to 7 cycles per second, called *theta waves,* after Berger's use of Greek letters. In stage 1 sleep, also known as the "drowsy state," you are no longer strongly aware of your surroundings, even though you may feel awake. (Stage 1 sleep is designated "drowsy" by sleep-lab technicians, possibly because about half the people who show a stage 1 reading on the polygraph say, if asked, that they are awake.) Your thoughts drift, and you may start to have dreamlike reveries.

Falling deeper into sleep, you next enter stage 2, or "medium" sleep. The EEG looks much less regular now. Voltage and frequency vary greatly compared to the earlier stage of sleep. The large, slow waves of deep sleep begin to be seen. Sleep "spindles" appear on the paper—rapid bursts of activity measuring some 12 to 14 cycles per second and lasting half a second or a bit longer. These are never found during normal wakefulness.

About 30 to 45 minutes after falling asleep, the EEG output seems to be composed almost entirely of big, mountainous humps. These are called *delta waves* or slow waves, and they signify delta sleep or slow-wave sleep. The frequency of these slow waves is 1 to 3 cycles per second. The frenetic activity of billions of neurons engaged in the tasks of wakefulness has long disappeared, allowing large, slow deflections of the pen. When the pages written by the polygraph pens show 20 percent slow waves, sleep is defined as stage 3. When slow waves account for 50 percent of the polygraph readings, then stage 4 has been reached.

During sleep, heart rate and blood pressure gradually fall to their lowest values in the 24-hour period, except during dreaming sleep, when they fluctuate as in wakefulness. Breathing slows down as well. The brain cools off during delta sleep: its temperature is reduced and the cerebral blood flow diminishes, probably because the higher levels of the brain are used less intensively during deep sleep. Delta sleep often lasts for a solid period of half an hour or more. By the time the night is over, most people will have spent about 10 to 25 percent of their slumber in delta sleep.

Rapid eye movement (REM) sleep, or "dreaming" sleep, is just what its name implies. Your eyes are moving, possibly following dream images at times. In the REM stage, the body, except for the diaphragm and occasional muscle twitches, virtually ceases moving below the neck. It even relaxes its temperature regulation; you do not shiver in REM sleep, and your body temperature starts edging toward room temperature. Although your overall metabolism may be at a low point during REM sleep, brain activity picks up, and blood flow to the brain increases. Heart rate also fluctuates, as mentioned earlier. REM sleep generally begins about 90 minutes after the onset of sleep, although some individuals with "dream pressure" owing to distress, illness, or the use of or withdrawal from some drug may begin REM sleep less than an hour after falling asleep. Early appearing REM is thus a laboratory marker for trouble.

You drift between REM sleep and medium sleep (stage 2) for most of the night, but this is punctuated by dreaming periods during REM that appear perhaps three to five times, or about every 90 minutes. You probably dream every night, even if you are unable to remember the dreams when you wake up later. A certain amount of REM sleep seems to be necessary— about 20 percent of nightly sleep time in a typical adult. If human subjects are experimentally deprived of REM sleep for a night or two, the proportion of REM sleep rises sharply the following night, to perhaps 40 percent. Animal experiments suggest that REM sleep plays a role in storing learned information in memory.

REM sleep is neither deep nor light sleep as we commonly define those terms, although it shows features of both. For instance, at least as much noise is required to awaken a person from REM sleep as from stage 2 sleep; sometimes a similar amount of noise is needed to awaken someone from deep sleep. The REM sleeper is therefore not merely dozing. Even so, the mental activity of dreaming suggests that certain parts of the brain are extremely active and alert during REM sleep, and heart rate and blood pressure fluctuations are more like those of wakefulness. Because REM sleep seems to be neither light nor heavy sleep, most researchers think REM episodes ought to be put in a category of their own. Under that scheme, there are three basic states of the sleep-wake cycle: wakefulness, sleep, and the REM state.

Our understanding of the mechanisms of sleep is updated continually as researchers discover more and more information. By the 1930s, because of experimental incisions across the brain's axis at various levels, it was known that sleep and wakefulness were regulated in the lowest, most primitive levels of the brain. This makes sense: our sleep resembles that of our animal cousins, and at this level our brains show the most similarities with theirs. Research through the 1950s and 1960s focused on two particular lower-brain structures, the *locus coeruleus* ("blue place") and the *midline raphe* ("seam") *nuclei,* which have much to do with the regulation of sleep. The locus coeruleus is rich in the neurotransmitter noradrenaline and is connected with many brain structures that participate in REM sleep. Thus it sends impulses to nerve cells that move the eyes or inhibit the muscles, and also to nerve cells in the topmost layer of the nervous system, which becomes activated during REM sleep and possibly accounts for REM dreams.

The raphe nuclei are rich in serotonin and seem to regulate deep sleep; in animal experiments, deep sleep disappeared when the raphe nuclei were destroyed. Thus each of the two main types of sleep, REM and non-REM, has its own group of nerve cells. In the 1970s some researchers proposed a model to show how the alternation between the two basic types of sleep is controlled.

THE ON AND OFF SYSTEMS

This model postulates that two different brain systems are involved in generating REM sleep: an *on system* and an *off system*. The on system contains nerve cells that are most active during waking hours and reach a nadir of activity during REM sleep. The off system shows just the opposite pattern of activity. Its cells are busiest during REM sleep and are suppressed by the on system when we are awake. The on system involves neurons for which nerve signals are transmitted by noradrenaline, whereas the off system uses acetylcholine as a neurotransmitter. Thus, the constant alternation between dreaming, or REM sleep, and the other types of sleep—a continuum from light to deep sleep—is controlled by an oscillating system with its own structures and neurotransmitters.

As mechanisms for the regulation of sleep are further proposed and refined, some limitations in the models will still be present. Humans have qualitatively different nervous systems from even close animal relatives. In addition, we differ a great deal from one another neurologically and biochemically. We have a different nerve-cell profile and different proportions of different nerve cells, and we all have different levels of and sensitivities to neurotransmitters. Thus, the pictures researchers draw will show what is probable, rather than what is definite, for each individual.

Certain medications that work by changing the levels of neurotransmitters—such as some drugs for high blood pressure, asthma, depression, or heart-rhythm disturbances—also work more effectively for some people than others. Similarly, some people sleep well while taking such medications, while others do not. Even reliable drugs may have therapeutic effects in some people but not in others. Some antidepressant drugs decrease REM sleep significantly by increasing the action of noradrenaline. This effect may be therapeutic in some individuals, such as those who frequently have nightmares or breathe poorly during REM sleep, but may not help others with the same problems. This is why choosing medications for a particular patient is often more of an art than a science.

REM SLEEP AND DREAMS

Whatever its sources, and however controlled, REM sleep is the main dreaming period. Dreams may occur during other sleep stages, too, but as a rule our most significant dreams— those we recall upon awakening—take place in the REM sleep. When sleepers are awakened during periods of REM sleep, they describe dreams in vivid detail about 80 percent of the time. By contrast, if awakened during periods outside the REM episodes, they recall their dreams only about 20 percent of the time. Moreover, dreams reported from non-REM sleep are not so well formed; the sleeper might report sensations like colors or sounds, for example, rather than images and events.

Dreaming gives REM sleep a particular importance, because dreams may reflect or even help our mental and emotional well-being. The psychological theory of dreams was best discussed in the work of Sigmund Freud, who related what patients dreamed to their fears and unsolved problems. The bad dreams people have after experiencing traumatic events tend to confirm this idea. In dreams, people can soothe themselves with wished-for pleasures or try to deal with some of their own dark urges. This is the process that the Spanish portraitist Goya depicted in his famous etching of a man asleep at his desk. Behind him rises a swarm of grotesque winged beings representing his most fearsome dreams and instincts. The painting is captioned: "The sleep of reason produces monsters." Goya clearly understood the importance of sleep to mental health. Sleep is the time when we can deal best with many of the psychological problems that we must ignore or repress during our conscious, rational, waking hours.

Some contemporary theorists feel that dreams stimulate rather than reflect emotions. Not only do eye movements increase, but the organs of balance in the inner ear may also be stimulated, causing dreams of motion. Various theories about the causes of dreams lead to vastly different views on their meaning. Whereas one psychiatrist might interpret a dream of falling as psychologically important, depending on how the dreamer talks about it (the fall might symbolize a fall from grace or the fall that succeeds pride), another specialist might interpret the falling as the activation of certain brain stem nerve cells that ordinarily help maintain a person's orientation in space.

The biochemistry of sleep is only partially understood and the reasons for dreaming are open to speculation. Yet our knowledge of the sleep and dream processes, however incomplete, aids diagnosis and treatment of sleep disorders.

2
....

Insomnia and Narcolepsy: The Extremes of Sleep Disorders

DEFINING SLEEP DISORDERS

Sleep disorders come in many varieties, ranging from almost total sleeplessness to dreary, endless somnolence. Insomnia, however, is the most common sleep disorder. It can be caused by anything from poor light conditions to poor health. At the other extreme is excessive sleepiness, in which a person suffers either sudden attacks of sleep at inopportune times or continuous sleepiness. We will consider narcolepsy, a disease characterized by daytime sleepiness and brief sleep episodes, later.

Official classifications of sleep disorders have been made by both the American Sleep Disorders Association (ASDA) and the American Psychiatric Association (APA). The ASDA defines sleep disorders as "disturbed sleep." The APA defines them as disturbances "in the amount, timing, or quality of sleep" or "an abnormal event occurring during sleep." Sleep-disorders medicine is so new that definitions, terms, and concepts for sleep disorders are still being proposed. The newness of the field makes it difficult to state definitively who should determine the existence of a sleep disorder: the patient, the family, the doctor, or a laboratory test. Even if tests are made, the disorders that test findings can diagnose or rule out often remain in question. If a patient thinks he or she has disordered sleep, then he or she probably has it. The patient may not know exactly what is wrong but does know something is amiss.

But many sleep doctors do not agree with this approach. Some will monitor the sleep of an insomnia patient in the laboratory. If, as often happens, there are no signs of abnormal sleep in the record, they will tell the patient they can find nothing wrong. ASDA even has an official diagnosis for the situation: "sleep state misperception."

Furthermore, experiments have revealed that when awakened from the identical amount of sleep (as measured by a polygraph machine), people with insomnia will estimate they have slept much less compared with normal sleepers. This disparity between what insomnia patients say about their sleep and what the polygraph indicates poses a problem for researchers, who prefer objective data to confirm a patient's opinion. Those researchers contend that if you cannot objectively find some abnormal sleep, then nothing is wrong, at least with the sleep. However, there is another viewpoint: other researchers find that the objective-measurement view puts too much faith in the measurements of a machine, the output of which is limited to electrical signals, and that these signals may not explain everything about sleep and insomnia.

When some people complain of insomnia, their family members tell the doctor confidentially: "I heard him (or her) snoring for hours." A laboratory test may also indicate that the patient sleeps well. Nevertheless, the person complains. Possibly the sleep does not refresh the person enough, and the test did not detect what was actually wrong. Some people are sleepy all the time, but their families or teachers—or in some cases even the sufferers themselves—dismiss the problem as the product of a defective moral character. One drowsy patient, brought to the sleep clinic by his wife, said there was nothing wrong with him except "a lazy mind." Constant sleepiness, however, drains the color out of life; it is a problem even if no one recognizes it.

INSOMNIA: THE INABILITY TO SLEEP

Insomnia means that you wish to fall asleep but cannot. When terrible trauma or disappointment strikes, sleep may fail for a while. But the vexatious insomnia for which people seek help is the chronic kind, in which a person spends months or years in a futile quest for sound, refreshing sleep. Studies indicate that about 15 percent of Americans suffer from insomnia to some extent, and this figure increases to about 25 percent in people over 65.

Of course, insomnia is not the same in any two people. Some with insomnia suffer more than others. Publisher Joseph Pulitzer, for example, had such difficulty sleeping that he spent much of his time at sea on a specially soundproofed yacht where he could keep noise and other disturbances to a minimum. Many people with insomnia share Pulitzer's problem with noise. Yet noise does not always upset nor prevent sleep. You can become accustomed to loud noises and sleep through uproars that would awaken most others. A 1977 study of sleep patterns among residents living near the Los Angeles International Airport revealed the surprising result that most of them slept quite well.

Here are some other common causes of insomnia:

Artificial light. When Thomas Edison invented the electric light, he may not have realized his creation would keep millions of people awake nights in decades to come. Even had he known, he might not have worried much about it, since he himself needed only four or five hours of sleep each night. But the artificial light that enables us to stay up at night may also overturn our natural night-and-day sleep cycle. When the sun goes down, an internal "clock" (see chap. 3) signals it is time to sleep, but artificial light and the evening activities that go with it send a conflicting message that it is still wake time. If a person's hours of light vary greatly, as they can easily in a world full of light bulbs, the pacemakers that control the sleep/wake schedule may become confused and will not be able to determine whether it is time to sleep or not. The result can be troubled sleep or insomnia. Employees who work late at night or on rotating shifts are especially prone to insomnia from irregular "daytimes."

Migraines. Migraine headaches can be triggered during sleep, especially during dreaming sleep, which can stimulate production of adrenalinelike neurotransmitters that can set off a headache and rouse a person from sleep.

We know that some neurotransmitters have a hand in causing migraine pain because medications that relieve migraine tend to change levels of these substances. One prime suspect is serotonin, because some antiserotonin medications prevent migraine. Remarkably, some medications with the opposite physiological effect may also prevent migraine when antiserotonin medications do not work. This probably means that migraine headaches can derive from two biochemically opposite mechanisms. There may be some allergic mechanisms for migraine as well, or at least some substances that participate in the allergic reaction may also participate in the mechanisms for migraine. These substances are peptides, which are chains of amino acids, and are known as *neuropeptides* for their actions on the nervous system.

Drugs. Many drugs, from illicit compounds such as cocaine to prescription and over-the-counter medications, can interfere with sleep, but the most commonly used sleep-disrupting drugs are caffeine, alcohol, and nicotine (see chaps. 4 and 5). Caffeine, which can enter the diet in many ways, can interfere with sleep for 12 to 20 hours after you consume it. Nicotine is a strong, highly addicting stimulant that can also upset sleep. Although alcohol may make a person groggy enough to fall asleep, it actually disturbs sleep later. In short, the more drug-free your life is, the better you are likely to sleep.

Psychiatric problems. Not all psychiatric disorders interfere with sleep, but many do. Depression, anxiety, and other disorders may ruin sleep. Some psychiatric problems can set off a cycle of events that perpetuates insomnia for months or even years (see chap. 7).

Maladaptive behaviors. In their search for sound slumber, many insomnia sufferers inadvertently fall into bad habits that actually cost them sleep. Some try too hard to sleep and become so obsessed with it that the effort keeps them awake. Daytime naps may also produce poor sleep at night; periods of sleep, especially during the afternoon, can consume so much of the daily ration of deep sleep that the body feels less need to fall asleep at night.

Conditioned or "learned" wakefulness. People with a conditioned wakefulness problem have lain wide awake in their darkened bedrooms so often that they have come automatically to associate going to bed with sleeplessness. Their situation is like that of Pavlov's dog; they have been conditioned to link bedtime with wakefulness and discomfort. These antisleep associations can be overcome by reconditioning the insomnia sufferer into a less tense state.

Movement disorders. "Restless legs syndrome" is an example of a movement disorder that harms sleep. After retiring for the evening, some people suffer an agitated feeling deep in the legs, combined with twitches and other small leg movements when the legs are at rest. Mild pain and cramps may also occur, and sometimes it feels as if ants are crawling under the skin. This syndrome makes the individual feel an irresistible need to rise and walk around, thus destroying any chance of falling asleep. Restless legs syndrome may stem from affected nerves in the legs; diabetes or vitamin deficiencies may be involved, as may the effects of some drugs. Restless legs syndrome should not be confused with sleepwalking. Both conditions are discussed in chapter 10.

Disorders of the body. Disorders of all types can disrupt sleep. The pain from arthritic inflammation of large joints such as the hip and shoulder may interfere with sleep. Epilepsy can seriously affect sleep; twice the percentage of epilepsy patients report insomnia compared to the rest of the population. Asthmatic attacks can cause the sufferer to wake up in the middle of the night, gasping for air. Pain from digestive disorders such as peptic ulcers or hiatus hernias can keep one awake nights. So can cardiac troubles, including angina, a condition in which the heart muscle aches because it is not receiving enough oxygen through its own blood vessels, and prolapsed mitral valve syndrome, in which a heart valve abnormality is accompanied by increased sensitivities to adrenaline-like neurotransmitters that leave the would-be sleeper restless. Kidney and liver disorders may result in uremia, jaundice, or accumulations of other toxins in the body that impair functioning of the nervous system; this too can render a person sleepless.

Of course, some people do have problems with the actual sleep-making mechanisms of the nervous system. These people tend to have suffered with insomnia since childhood (see chap. 9) or to have some severe medical disorder. These types of problems are more likely to be treated in a sleep clinic. But even these problems can most often be remedied. Of 100 people with severe insomnia that were tracked in a study a few years ago, only 12 achieved insufficient relief, despite their earnest attempts. Today, because of more rapid progress in such a new field, probably most of them would find significant relief.

INSOMNIA CAUSED BY MOOD PROBLEMS AND A METABOLIC DISORDER

Quite often insomnia has multiple roots. Ms. D., a businesswoman and mother of two teenage sons, was 36 when she sought help in curing her insomnia. She had once been an energetic woman, but now she was prey to a deep depression and could barely meet her day-to-day obligations. Earlier when she had experienced dark moods, there usually had been a good reason for them. Now there was no reason for her depression, yet she felt worse than ever before. Ms. D. went to a sleep clinic for help because in addition to everything else, she had great difficulty sleeping. This condition, she said, had gone on for months.

Her physician at the clinic prescribed antidepressants for her mood and sleep problems. The antidepressants worked, but only up to a point. She slept a little better and felt more optimistic about dealing with life. But she still cried for long periods during her office visits. This crying suggested to her doctor that something was still wrong, because antidepressants usually bring near-total relief to patients who have functioned well previously and who have become severely depressed for no apparent reason. There seemed to be another underlying problem in Ms. D.'s case.

Both doctors and laypersons usually assume that a psychological symptom always has some psychological cause behind it, a correct assumption in many cases. But mind and body affect each other, and physiological changes can produce mental symptoms. If the cause of the psychological symptom is actually physiological, it may be easier to correct than a problem that is purely psychological. So Ms. D. underwent a set of blood screening tests to investigate her sleeplessness and depression.

In her case, the tests paid off. They indicated she had a problem with her thyroid gland, which secretes hormones that help govern the rate at which the body metabolizes food. Ms. D. showed low levels of *thyroxine,* a thyroid hormone, but high levels of *thyroid-stimulating hormone* (TSH) that is secreted by the pituitary gland, a pea-size, vital organ underneath the brain. The pituitary gland had reacted to Ms. D.'s low level of thyroxine by putting out more and more TSH to "stoke" the thyroid gland back up to its proper level of activity. Normally, this self-corrective procedure acts through a feedback loop, like a reciprocating control between two instruments such as a furnace and thermostat. High levels of TSH signal the thyroid to increase production of thyroxine, which signals the pituitary gland to slow down production of TSH, and vice versa.

Unfortunately, the feedback loop wasn't working in this case. Try as it might, the pituitary gland was unable to stimulate the thyroid to produce enough thyroxine. Something appeared to be limiting production of thyroid hormones, leaving the body with insufficiently low levels. When that happens, the thyroid gland is usually diseased. Sometimes *antibodies*—disease-fighting molecules that the body produces to ward off infection—are involved. Aberrant antibodies can be produced that attack tissues of the body itself, as happens in autoimmune diseases. In this case, Ms. D. was producing antibodies that tended to destroy her own thyroid tissues. Those antibodies showed up clearly in follow-up blood tests.

Thus, the causes of Ms. D.'s woes were complex. In addition to depression, she had a familial condition called *Hashimoto's thyroiditis*. Thyroid hormone normally helps the action of nervous system neurotransmitters. Neurotransmitters together with metabolic rate, as controlled by thyroid hormone, profoundly affect sleep. Thus, the chemical battle being waged in her body against her own thyroid tissues had deprived Ms. D. of sleep, energy, and emotional stability. That was why antidepressants had inadequate effect on her insomnia problem.

Ms. D. started taking thyroid hormone replacement pills while she remained on the antidepressant medication. Soon all her symptoms vanished. She slept well and resumed her normal activities. Although she had to remain on the thyroid replacement medication, Ms. D. was able to discontinue the antidepressants after a year.

Thyroid hormone stimulates the action of neurotransmitter substances that regulate sleep. Therefore any disease that causes too much or too little thyroid hormone, such as hyperthyroidism, drug suppression of the thyroid, lack of iodine to make thyroid hormone, or primary hypothyroidism, can worsen sleep. Other hormones influence sleep as well, and problems with the glands that produce them, such as diseases of the adrenal gland or the pituitary gland, can cause insomnia. These hormonal or *endocrine* problems exemplify how sleep is a general health barometer that can reflect chronic medical conditions and can sometimes be the first sign of them.

NARCOLEPSY

Narcolepsy usually begins in adolescence or the early adult years as an insidious increase in naps and sleepiness. It progresses to the point where the sufferer has sudden, unexpected, and irresistible urges to sleep at various times of day. Narcolepsy victims may find it difficult to drive, sit through a movie, or read a book without dozing off. Sometimes they also have attacks of sudden, temporary weakness. They may get so weak in the knees that they slump to the floor. Often these incidents occur during sudden bouts of emotion, especially laughter, anger, or surprise. After a few moments, they can stand up again.

These patients are so sleepy that one diagnostic test for narcolepsy measures how fast a person falls asleep. This is called the Multiple Sleep Latency Test, originally devised at the Stanford Sleep Disorders Center. In this test, a person simply lies down on a comfortable bed in the sleep lab and is hooked up to a polygraph. The lights are turned out, the technician closes the door, and the time needed to fall asleep is measured. Technicians ask the patient to lie down and nap four or five times during a day, usually every two hours, beginning at about 10:00 A.M. Remarkably, on the average nap, patients with narcolepsy fall asleep in less than five minutes (see fig. 2). Furthermore, they tend to have REM sleep soon after the onset of sleep, unlike most people, in whom REM sleep first appears 70 to 100 minutes after the onset of sleep. This swift appearance of REM sleep might cause the narcolepsy symptoms described below. Remember that in REM sleep, except for the diaphragm, we are more or less paralyzed from the neck down and we dream. The symptoms of narcolepsy include sudden muscle weakness as well as hallucinations or "dreams" suddenly intruding outside of their normal sleep times, as if REM sleep had suddenly appeared during wakefulness.

Another symptom of narcolepsy is automatic behavior, the repetition of tasks that starts out with a purpose, such as cleaning a room or wrapping a package, but that can go on for half an hour or more without the person being aware of what he or she is doing. (Automatic behavior does not necessarily mean a person has narcolepsy. Other sleepy people experience automatic behavior at one time or another, notably conscientious people who try to work even when too tired.)

Some symptoms of narcolepsy are harrowing. A narcoleptic may awaken suddenly in the night, feeling frightened, and find that he or she is totally paralyzed, unable to move for what seems an hour or more, although the actual time elapsed is usually less than a minute. Hallucinations also affect the narcolepsy sufferer, who may see things just before falling asleep

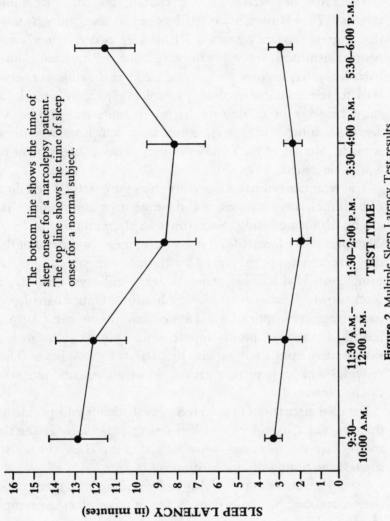

The bottom line shows the time of sleep onset for a narcolepsy patient. The top line shows the time of sleep onset for a normal subject.

Figure 2 Multiple Sleep Latency Test results.

or feel another person's presence in the room when he or she is really all alone. Fortunately, the person with narcolepsy usually distinguishes between the hallucinations and reality.

The cause of narcolepsy is unknown, but there are some theories. The abnormality of REM sleep is clear, and we know that a great tendency toward REM sleep occurs when some neurotransmitters, especially noradrenaline, are depleted. Thus, narcolepsy may involve some abnormality in the ability of nerve cells to release noradrenaline. Narcolepsy patients also show some evidence of an abnormally low manufacture and use of *dopamine,* another neurotransmitter from which noradrenaline is made. Studies of the families of narcolepsy patients point to a possible genetic link.

The treatment of narcolepsy involves purposeful scheduling of bedtimes, arising times, and daytime naps in a routine that can be maintained daily. Sometimes an afternoon nap of 15 or 20 minutes may forestall significant sleepiness for the rest of the day. Some patients may need more than one nap daily or, if being treated with drugs, naps on drug "holidays" (one day a week on which patients take no medication). Until a narcolepsy patient achieves optimal wakefulness, he or she must keep a record of when symptoms appear, what they were, his or her sleep pattern, and anything else that affects the condition. This provides a baseline picture against which therapeutic progress can be measured.

Detailed discussions of such records can identify the problems that worsen a narcolepsy patient's sleepiness, such as certain meals, exercise, meetings, or other activities. The records also suggest the timing of any medication regime.

Some patients with narcolepsy can get along with predictable sleep scheduling plus daily naps. A few others prefer their symptoms to taking medication. For most patients, however, some drug treatment is needed. Many narcolepsy patients are diagnosed by a doctor who immediately prescribes drugs, most often stimulants, and thereafter treats them with automatic refills of the drugs. This tends to relieve those patients with milder forms of the disease. For those less easily remedied, more work is needed, such as schedule keeping and working out a sleep and nap regimen, which require careful examination of daily records.

For patients with milder narcolepsy, treatment with stimulants often reverses the problem. Caffeine and caffeinated beverages are sometimes useful, but the caffeine dose must be standardized by taking the exact same dose of the same form at the same time daily, down to the details of using the same brand, and percolating, drip brewing, or steeping the coffee or tea in the same way. Stimulants such as methylphenidate (Ritalin) and dextroamphetamine (Dexadrine) now have a poor reputation because they were abused as weight-loss pills in the 1950s and as euphoria makers in the 1960s, which led to strict laws concerning their use. Pharmacists have questioned customers about these stimulants, or have indicated that a prescription for one of these drugs is not routine. Actually, these drugs have an excellent safety record when used responsibly. Often they continue to work consistently if the patient takes a drug "holiday" one day a week. Pemoline (Cylert) is a longer-acting drug that does not have harsh laws attached to it. These stimulants probably increase the actions of dopamine, the neurotransmitter that does not function normally in narcolepsy patients.

Patients with narcolepsy who experience cataplexy (collapsing when excited), bad dreams, or hallucinations at the onset of sleep are often relieved by antidepressants. These drugs increase the actions of noradrenaline, which lessen REM sleep–related symptoms. Cataplexy, hallucinations, and bad dreams—and sleep paralysis as well—probably represent the unnatural intrusion of REM sleep, or at least parts of it, into wakefulness. Antidepressants can increase the neurotransmitters that decrease the amount of REM sleep.

NARCOLEPSY TREATED WITH MEDICATION

Narcolepsy treatment often involves schedule and medication adjustments. Ms. C., a 40-year-old assistant to a stockbroker, had been excessively sleepy for about 25 years when she finally sought help. She usually went to bed about 11:00 P.M. each night, waking up around 5:00 A.M. for a 90-minute drive to work. Her somewhat short six-hour sleep schedule aggravated her symptoms. When asleep, she had frequent dreams and occasional nightmares. Once she was up, she had trouble staying awake, and operating a car was especially difficult for her. A few times she had hallucinations while driving along in a drowsy condition.

One day she fell asleep at the wheel, and her car left the road and careened down an embankment. Fortunately, Ms. C. climbed out unhurt and was able to make her way up the embankment. Shaken, she went soon afterward to see a neurologist who put her on medication he hoped would improve the quality of her sleep. But her problems continued, and she sought advice from a sleep clinic.

Ms. C. was obviously depressed, and depression occurs frequently in people with narcolepsy. Although a battery of tests failed to absolutely confirm the diagnosis, Ms. C.'s hallucinations strongly indicated narcolepsy, and she was prescribed an antidepressant that worked well at first. Ms. C. showed no further symptoms, except that she sometimes felt the need for a nap at lunchtime, which she would take.

New problems arose when Ms. C. was assigned to work with another broker. He was aggressive, demanding, and propositioned her sexually. In addition to the distress her new boss caused, Ms. C. had to attend lengthy meetings during the lunch hour when she was accustomed to taking a nap. She also began studying for professional accreditation at an evening course that met twice a week. Her narcoleptic problems with driving began to recur. One time she reached into her pocket for her car keys and was startled to find a cold lump of cheese instead. At the moment of her surprise, she suddenly felt weak all over and she fell to the ground.

Ms. C.'s troubles show what the narcoleptic patient must overcome: Work can be scheduled just at the wrong time, or emotional reactions can cause symptoms to return. Ms. C. had frequent discussions with her doctor to figure out how to cope with the changes that had caused the symptoms to return. Discussions focused on how she could master her current conditions. She then requested a transfer to another department. A stimulant was added to her drug regimen to be taken prior to the nighttime lectures. Her sleep records revealed that she stayed up too late each evening, paradoxically becoming too tired and disorganized to prepare for bed.

Ms. C. took a regularly scheduled vacation and found that most of her problems vanished, and she concluded that her sleep schedule and troublesome boss provoked most of her symptoms. She returned from vacation determined to control her narcolepsy, and eventually she increased her nightly sleep hours. Fortunately she did acquire a new supervisor, which relieved much of the pressure on her. She no longer had sleep attacks while driving, and moved forward in her work and social life.

Narcolepsy has specific symptoms, especially sleepiness, but it affects all of a person's life. Its causes are unknown, although neurotransmitter abnormalities that bring on REM sleep at unusual times may be an underlying factor. Milder forms can be treated effectively by sleep scheduling or drug use alone; more difficult cases require a careful review of sleep records and progressive refinement of scheduling and drug regimens. Narcoleptics have formed an advocacy group to help sufferers, educate the public, and to raise research funds. The American Narcolepsy Association may be contacted at P.O. Box 1187, San Carlos, California 98070. The Narcolepsy Network emphasizes support groups and is reached at P.O. Box 1365, FDR Station, New York, New York 10150.

RECOGNIZING SLEEP DISORDERS

The case histories of Ms. D. and Ms. C. show that even severe cases of sleep disorders can be treated successfully, but first someone must recognize the problems. Sleep disorders, however, can be hard to recognize. A person who sleeps too much may not consider the problem an illness, or even a problem at all. Sleepiness is not like an itch or a pain that compels people to notice it. On the contrary, people often ignore subtler signs of disease such as a cough or palpitations—because indicators like these do not convey the same urgency as severe pain and fever.

It is the same with sleepiness. Many individuals just explain away their sleepiness by a heavy workload, even if their families or their doctors raise questions. Some people make an appointment at a sleep clinic only after a traffic accident or near miss convinces them that excessive sleepiness is serious.

Insomnia patients complain far more than those who suffer from excessive sleepiness or sleep disorders such as sleepwalking or bad dreams. Yet surveys show that most people who have sleep problems do not receive treatment for it—they simply do not go to doctors for help.

Perhaps their reluctance is a holdover from the not-too-distant past, when doctors knew little about sleep disorders and were limited in their ability to help a patient cope with them. For example, sleep apnea, the condition in which the sleeper stops breathing for frequent short periods during the night (see chap. 10), was unrecognized 25 years ago. Narcolepsy, though known for a century, was largely neglected by the medical profession, and insomnia of all kinds was often dismissed as anxiety and treated with sleeping pills.

Today, however, doctors increasingly recognize sleeplessness as an actual symptom of potentially serious medical conditions. They now consider chronic insomnia a red flag indicating many conditions that need detailed investigation and treatment. The doctor's understanding is reflected in medical statistics: Use of sleeping pills in the United States fell almost 40 percent during the 1970s as doctors realized that these pills do not relieve most insomnia in the long run.

If you often get less sleep than you feel you need, if you frequently have trouble falling asleep, if you feel too sleepy during the day, or if you suffer from any other discomforting problem related to sleep, you have a sleep disorder worth discussing with a physician (see chaps. 11 and 12).

3

·············

The "Sleep Clock" and Its Disorders

Night and sleep go together. A natural body "clock" that is part of our evolutionary heritage governs our daily sleep/wake cycle. This clock affects us when we sleep and when we awaken. Ordinarily it keeps us asleep at night and awake during the day, in a 24-hour cycle of sleeping and wakefulness known as a circadian rhythm (from the Latin *circa,* about, and *dies,* day). There are also circadian rhythms governing vital functions such as body temperature, hormone secretion, enzyme production, and electrolyte excretion; all of these functions increase and decrease over the course of a day. The worth of these rhythms to the human organism may lie in adapting us to daytime activity and nighttime rest. All organisms display circadian rhythms, and it seems reasonable to assume that circadian rhythms aid survival (see chap. 1).

Circadian rhythms may increase the efficiency of an organism by making enzyme production efficient. Enzymes are complex molecules and require a great deal of energy to assemble. Certain rhythms "schedule" enzyme secretion for moments when the enzymes are most likely to have *substrates,* the substances they work on, available. The conversion of the neurotransmitter dopamine to noradrenaline, which was mentioned in connection with narcolepsy mechanisms, depends on an enzyme called *dopamine hydroxylase.* Thus dopamine is the substrate for the enzyme. If enzyme levels peaked at a time when they did not have optimal amounts of substrate to engage, some of the energy needed to make the enzymes would be wasted. Organisms trying to survive in a competitive environment cannot afford to waste energy, and thus circadian rhythms that make enzyme production efficient help ensure the survival of the individual and the species.

Circadian rhythms, however, are not the only kind of biological cycle that governs our lives. There are also 90-minute rhythms that influence when we are most, and least, efficient on the job. Other rhythms affect children and determine the time they are most apt to stage tantrums; still other rhythms regulate when adults are most likely to display electroencephalographic patterns indicating a lack of alertness. Menstruation in women is a function of monthly rhythms. And there are even studies that point to some yearly rhythms: One French researcher has noted a peak in February for death rates due to stroke. The same researcher observed that May signals a low point in the excretion of male hormones, and he determined that children's intake of fats and carbohydrates decreased in winter, while intake of proteins decreased in summer. One researcher and his wife had their urine tested daily for 16 years and found 5-year rhythms for electrolyte excretion.

The circadian cycle is not fixed immutably, and numerous factors can change it. Sometimes events knock our circadian rhythms out of control and make us sleep at unusual and inconvenient moments. Some people find themselves compelled to sleep from 2:00 A.M. to 9:00 A.M., even though earlier sleep and awakening would get them to work on time. Fortunately, disorders involving circadian rhythms usually can be remedied. The therapy may involve resetting the internal clock. To do this, you may have to set yourself a regular time to get up each morning, because rising time helps regulate the length of circadian cycles.

EXAMPLES OF CIRCADIAN RHYTHMS IN ACTION

A familiar example of an organism that shows circadian rhythm is the mimosa, a small flowering tree whose delicate, featherlike leaves have a peculiar property: at night they close, folding down the middle like a shut book. In the morning, the leaves open again. The leaves behave as if they were sensitive to light or temperature so the mimosa came to be called the "sensitive plant."

Among the first scientists to observe this leaf-closing phenomenon was the French astronomer Jean-Jacques de Mairan, whose interests were not confined to the heavens. He also was intrigued by biology, and especially by the circadian rhythm of the mimosa.

How, de Mairan asked himself, did the mimosa know when to open and shut its leaves? Were the leaves merely responding somehow to the presence or absence of sunlight, or did the mimosa have an internal timer of some kind that kept it in synchrony with the daily cycle of light and darkness? To find out, de Mairan devised a simple experiment. He put a mimosa inside a darkened shed for several days and went inside at regular intervals to observe it, taking care not to let in enough sunlight to trigger any light-induced reflexes the plant might have. What he found astonished him. Even when deprived of sunlight for 24 hours at a stretch, the mimosa's leaves kept opening and closing on schedule, as if the plant were still standing in the open.

The mimosa, de Mairan wrote, did not have to be standing outdoors for its leaves to open and shut; the plant's leaves "still [open] . . . markedly in the daytime and . . . [close] regularly in the evening, for the whole night. In this way, the sensitive plant senses the sun without seeing it in any way." De Mairan was wrong to say the plant senses the sunlight and responds accordingly. Incoming sunlight does not induce the leaves to open immediately. They are timed by a circadian rhythm of the plant itself, a preexisting cycle that the hours of sunlight adjust toward longer or shorter periods.

This circadian timing is common to many other plants,

though their rhythms may not be the same. Different flowers open at different times of the day. European gardeners in the eighteenth century took advantage of the individual circadian rhythms of flowers to create a kind of garden called the flower clock. In this garden about a dozen species of flowers were planted, arranged in individual beds that formed a clock face. Each species opened or closed approximately one hour after the one before it on the clock. Marigolds would open about 7:00 A.M., hawkweeds around 8:00 A.M., and so forth. In the afternoon, other flowers would mark the hours by their times of closing, finishing around 6:00 P.M. with the shutting of the primrose. Flower clocks may still be seen in some American and European gardens, elegant evidence of nature's circadian rhythms.

COMPONENTS OF A BIOLOGICAL CLOCK

It appears that we have two biological clocks that are usually synchronized with each other, because of the simultaneous, daily rise and fall of various functions in the human body, such as temperature. We believe there are two clocks, because if an animal is kept in constant light or constant darkness, or if a person is confined in an unchanging environment without knowing what time of day it is, the normally synchronized bodily rhythms start to break apart. For instance, the body-temperature rhythm, like all other daily rhythms, normally shows one long up-and-down cycle every 24 hours. The sleep/wake rhythm is similar, with one long wake period and sleep period, or sleep/wake cycle, per 24 hours. But under conditions in which the individual suddenly has no clue about the time of day, these rhythms become disconnected from each other.

One volunteer living in a time-cue-free laboratory developed a body-temperature rhythm with a 24.5-hour cycle, accompanied by a separate sleep/wake rhythm with a 33-hour cycle. He slept once every 33 hours, instead of once every 24, but his body temperature rose and fell very close to the usual 24-hour cycle. In isolation experiments, everyone desynchronizes eventually in this manner if the experiment lasts long enough. (Mysteriously, this will happen more quickly in neurotic individuals.) People in this desynchronized state may feel unwell and complain of a generalized "blah" feeling.

In figure 3 you can see what happens to the sleep schedule of someone who is kept unaware of the time of day. This is a volunteer living in a specially constructed underground laboratory, where there are no watches, radios, calendars, newspaper deliveries, or anything else that tells a person what time it is. In the experiment, the volunteer arises at about the same time each day until day 5, when his schedule starts moving later by about one hour each day. After day 8, the schedule shifts later much faster, at the rate of nine hours each day. This relates to the normal tendency of some people, especially the young, to move sleep times to slightly later hours, which makes a person stay up beyond a regular bedtime or sleep later on vacations. Such a tendency can be seen as a regular, progressive delay of the sleep schedule. It is difficult to define the schedule of the biological clocks and whether a person's rhythms are indeed synchronized, but people who go to bed progressively later or earlier may disrupt the synchronization of their clocks and might suffer some worsening of sleep quality.

Notice also that the rhythm of body temperature does not adapt to the new schedule. The lowest temperature for the 24-hour day normally comes toward the end of the night, just before it begins to rise in preparation for daytime. But the temperature rhythm continues to move with the slightly longer 24.5-hour schedule. As a result, the day's minimum temperature edges back from late night and is now reached in the middle of the day. Unfortunately, people are generally less alert when they reach their minimum body temperature; they don't perform tasks well either. Volunteers in experiments have shown a peak in task errors at around 4:00 A.M., when body temperature is lowest. Accident rates peak at around four in the morning, as well. The nuclear power plant accidents at Three Mile Island and at Chernobyl occurred around this time.

Throughout such experiments, one finding stands out: circadian rhythms operate under only two timetables, and there-

The solid lines show activity time, the dotted lines show rest time. Circles show minimal daily body temperature. The open circles drawn from day 10 indicate minimum body temperature corrected for 24 or 48 hours (true circadian periods) while the solid circles show, throughout the subject's time in the laboratory, the changes in the relationship between minimum body temperature and activity cycle.

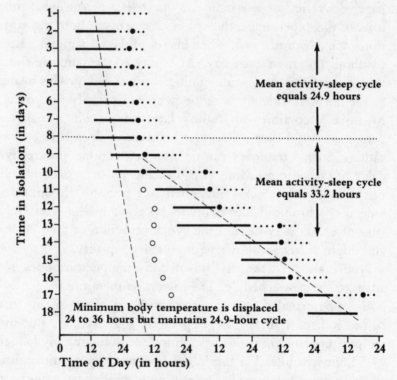

Figure 3 Free-running circadian rhythm in a human subject in an underground laboratory without any time cues.

fore only two timing systems seem to be present. One timing system governs body temperature and another governs the sleep/wake cycle, for example. Sleep researchers have never found more than two completely unrelated timetables in the same individual.

Biological clocks depend on external pacemakers to signal to them what time it is in the outside world. In plants and most animals, the principal pacemaker is the cycle of light and darkness produced by sunrise and sunset. For humans, however, another pacemaker is involved and frequently more important: the social schedule. The daily rhythm of one's social life does as much, if not more, than sunrise and nightfall to keep our biological clocks timed on a near-24-hour schedule. The social schedule may take many forms, from a daily wake-up call at 7:00 A.M., to a child waking you up early every morning, to watching late-night television regularly. Work schedules and regular mealtimes also contain timing information that helps keep body functions regulated and properly synchronized.

Many of our social schedules now deviate considerably from the light/dark cycle, because much social activity takes place by artificial light. But artificial light fails to impress very much our internal "timer," which was coded by ages of evolution to respond to the much brighter light of the sun. If a person has little exposure to the intensity of light outdoors, the natural day/night cycle may start to lose its pacemaking influence, and in its absence that person's rhythms may be thrown off course or become desynchronized. We will see shortly how this can damage sleep.

In countries of the far north, prolonged winter nights require people to spend even more of their waking time in artificial light. But, as mentioned, for many people light/dark cycles in which the light is mostly artificial are not sufficient to provide timing information for internal clocks. These people thus become like subjects in isolation experiments who do not really know the time of day. Little clinical research has been done on the internal-clock functions of those who suffer insomnia, but it is likely that some people are more sensitive than others to external pacemakers such as the light/dark cycle or social schedule. And people who are less sensitive might have more trouble with their internal clocks and be more likely to become desynchronized. This would interfere with their sleep cycles if, for example, their body temperature or adrenal hormone rhythms were rising when they went to bed; declining rhythms and temperature are the norm at bedtime.

The importance of sunrise and sunset is also apparent in individuals who respond little to social interaction, such as hospitalized schizophrenic patients. Because they often avoid people, the natural daily cycle of night and day becomes their strongest pacemaker.

Where in the body are these clocks located? Most evidence points to the brain. The brain's main job is to negotiate between the needs of the body and the demands of the outside world. As part of that task, the clocks help the body adapt to the constant changes in the light/dark cycle. One of these clocks appears to be located in a specific group of nerve cells (or nucleus) of the hypothalamus, a complex set of nuclei at the base of the brain that coordinates many vital functions. Experiments on animals have shown that when the superchiasmic nucleus (see p. 10) is removed from the hypothalamus, some body rhythms, such as the rest/activity cycle, may break down and be replaced by a random, unpredictable pattern of activity rather than a rhythmical one. Thus, it will be difficult to predict the times a laboratory guinea pig will decide to exercise on its running wheel. Yet other rhythms, such as the rise and fall of body temperature, will persist even in the absence of this nucleus. There must be another built-in pacemaker for temperature and other body functions, but the location of such a "temperature clock" has yet to be found.

On a more fundamental level, rhythmical timing is a basic function of life, down to individual cells. Cells grown in tissue culture and deprived of input from the nervous system exhibit regular schedules for physiological functions, such as secretion of enzymes. Single-celled plants also show predictable timing in their body functions, even when they are removed from all external sources of timing information, such as sunlight. How could such isolated, individual cells be able to time their functions? They must have a clock. Research suggests that this clock is located in the nucleus of the cell. But wherever an organism's internal clock resides, timing is at the root of all life, and features consistently shared between plants and animals must be at the very center of life processes. Metabolism is one of these features common to both plants and animals. The biological clocks are another. The laws of these physiological timing systems seem constant across not only species and phyla, but across the entire plant and animal kingdoms as well. Thus, timing seems central to life.

DESYNCHRONIZATION AND ADJUSTMENT

Ordinarily, all the circadian rhythms of the human body are tied together in a cycle about 24 hours long. Thus, a typical person with a regular schedule is probably asleep at 3:30 A.M., with heart rate and temperature at a low point, and the person's level of performance probably would be poor if he or she were awakened and asked to perform some sophisticated mental work. By 8:00 A.M., the typical person is probably awake and reasonably alert. Every hour of the day, the person has slightly different mental and physiological activity profiles, so time of day is an important factor in interpreting these measurements. A body temperature of 98.8° F. at 8:00 A.M. may indicate a slight fever, whereas the same temperature measured in late afternoon is consistent with good health.

For all of our body's functions to ebb and flow in a properly coordinated manner, the sleep/wake cycle and body-temperature cycle must be synchronized. As we saw in figure 3, however, some of these functions can get out of synchrony with one another. In the figure, temperature, which represents many metabolic processes, rises and falls out of synchrony with the sleep/wake cycle. Poor sleep is likely to result, because sleep is best under a slowing metabolic rate. But the rhythms of enzymes and substrates mentioned earlier also become uncoordinated.

Powerful conservatism underlies the basic processes of life: the main principle that organizes behavior is survival, and therefore vital processes are redundantly controlled to assure it. Modern contrivances, such as artificial light or jet aircraft, can make sudden changes in the light/dark cycle, but the body's clocks will adjust only gradually, and its physiological economy will be strained during such an adjustment period. Thus, many different factors can upset the internal timers. An erratic work schedule can do it, as can an arctic winter or jet travel from one time zone to another.

When timing information grows insufficient, a peculiar thing happens. Deprived of regular daily settings or signals, body clocks manifest periods slightly longer than 24 hours, a phenomenon known as free running. In the case where a person without external timing information developed a temperature rhythm of 24.5 hours and a sleep/wake rhythm of 33 hours, the rhythms were running free, unconstrained by external timing influences.

Few measurements of these rhythms have ever been obtained on persons suffering from sleep problems, but we know that many sleep disorders result when timing information is chaotic, variable, or insufficient. Maddeningly unpredictable sleep patterns may be the result of conflicts between other sleep regulators and the body's clock. An individual who lacked sleep previously may try to doze off at times when his or her body's metabolism is increasing—that is, preparing for wakefulness and activity—rather than decreasing. Sleep in this case represents a fight against an internal environment that is geared up for work or play rather than rest. Human metabolism tends toward normal levels for wakefulness, not toward sleep. Sleep then becomes a compromise, rather than a coordination, between sleep regulators at work in the brain. As soon as sleep becomes lighter, as it normally does after the first hour or two, the individual may well wake up instead of proceeding toward more refreshing slumber.

THE HUMAN CIRCADIAN SLEEP RHYTHM

Actual sleep rhythms are not perfectly steady because no biological rhythm is absolutely regular and because a little flexibility
in your sleep rhythm can be a distinct advantage. In some situations, sleepiness is inappropriate. Humans must then override
the circadian-rhythm-based urge to sleep for a while, until a
safer or more convenient time for sleep arrives.

How flexible is our circadian sleep cycle? Experiments in the
United States and Great Britain have provided some answers.
One Englishman spent more than 100 days underground in a cave
and kept track of his sleep schedule. He found that his circadian
cycle of sleep and wakefulness stretched out slightly. Eventually
his timing system, deprived of external timing information,
reverted to its own inherent, longer cycle, about 25 hours.

In 1938, two Americans, Nathaniel Kleitman and Bruce Richardson of the University of Chicago, performed an experiment
to see if they could readjust their biological clocks from a 24-
hour daily cycle to 28 hours. They secluded themselves in a
chamber at Mammoth Cave, Kentucky, and tried to force themselves into a specific pattern: 9 hours of sleep and 19 hours of
wakefulness.

Richardson succeeded. He was only in his early twenties, so
for him the readjustment was fairly easy, and he slipped into
the 28-hour cycle in a little over a week. But Kleitman, in his
forties, failed because he was older and therefore more susceptible to desynchronization of his internal systems. During the
day he was drowsy and grumpy, and at night he had trouble
falling asleep. The same unpleasant experiences can affect anyone who departs too much from a regular 24-hour sleep/wake
cycle. This may induce sleepiness in the middle of the day or
wakefulness in the middle of the night.

JET LAG

The phenomenon of jet lag is familiar to many who have taken
a cross-country or overseas airplane flight. After a flight from

New York to Honolulu, the traveler finds him- or herself on Hawaiian time, but his or her circadian rhythms are still set to New York time, a difference of some eight to nine hours. So this hypothetical traveler may have trouble staying up until Hawaiian bedtime in Honolulu, because the body is used to retiring much earlier. The resulting out-of-sync sleep schedule, and the various problems that accompany it, is commonly called *jet lag.* When travel is slower, by passenger ship or cross-country train, there is more time to reset the sleep clock. But jet aircraft, like artificial lights, have no regard for our circadian rhythms.

Jet lag takes longer to overcome after some flights than others. Generally, traveling east is more disruptive to sleep than traveling west, because our internal clocks, as mentioned earlier, tend toward operating on a slightly-longer-than-24-hour day unless directed otherwise by external signals. With this natural tendency to lengthen the body's day, we are inclined to get up and to go to bed later and later, rather than earlier.

Dr. Franz Halberg is a chronobiologist, a scientist who studies biological rhythms. He once measured body-temperature rhythms in a group of his colleagues in Minneapolis traveling to and from a conference in Japan. Halberg discovered that his group needed only eight days to conform with local time after arrival in Japan but almost two weeks to readjust when they were back in Minneapolis.

The reason is the sun's apparent motion across the sky as the earth rotates on its axis. The sun appears to rise in the east and set in the west, and thus the travelers moved with the sun on the way west, but opposite to the sun on the flight home. The scientists' systems found it harder to resume their former temperature rhythm when they got back to the United States; the day seemed to end too early, and their body clocks had a hard time adjusting (body clocks tend to schedule sleep for later hours).

If you are planning a long-distance flight on work or vacation, jet lag need not concern you greatly if you are flying a few hours westward. Your own body clocks naturally tend to set themselves later so that you will move gradually toward local time after a few days of getting up earlier. Should you be flying more than a few hours eastward, however, you may wish to alter your schedule gradually before you leave, to bring yourself more into line with the local time and schedule at your destination. If you are flying to a city where local time is six hours earlier than at home, you might try going to bed 10 minutes earlier every other night starting five weeks prior to the trip. This adjustment will reset your sleep time about three hours earlier, at a gradual pace that your other internal rhythms can keep up with. Thus you will have a head start in adjusting to the change of daily schedule.

If you start later than five weeks prior to your trip, or your social schedule will not permit you a bedtime three hours earlier, even a partial readjustment might help. All this might seem too much trouble for the tourist who arrives in Paris at noon (6:00 A.M. body time), simply takes a nap or goes to bed early, and pushes him- or herself through any sleepiness the next day. The daytime sleepiness occurs because the tourist left his or her body-temperature rhythm in New York. The temperature rhythm still reaches a low-temperature point at 4:00 A.M. New York time, which is 10:00 A.M. Paris time. And the tourist is likely to have a low temperature, and thus feel drowsy and unenergetic, at about 10:00 A.M. for a few days until the temperature—moving slowly in accord with the stately pace of the basic life processes—gradually readjusts to Paris time.

Of course, the adjustment seems too slow and arduous for many travelers, who decide to take sleeping pills to force a sleep/wake schedule consistent with their destinations. Triazolam (Halcion) is a popular drug, since research reports suggest that it can force the sleep/wake cycle to change faster. However, three neuroscientists once unknowingly had about a 10-hour period of amnesia after they flew to Europe taking triazolam en route. This gave rise to a condition they described as "traveler's amnesia." They remembered none of the events of the first 10 hours—arriving in Europe, having meals, and meeting with colleagues. Amnesia would seem to be a heavy price to pay to lessen the effects of jet lag.

To summarize, the body's clock adjusts more slowly than

jets can travel. The more you gradually adjust to the schedule of your destination, the less jet lag you suffer. Eastward flights, moving sleep earlier and against the underlying tendency of our clocks toward later bedtimes, are harder to adjust to than westward flights.

As with most sleep problems, one person's jet lag may be much different from another's. Jet lag affects young people and short sleepers less. Many people are only mildly affected. If you suffer from insomnia or have other sleep problems, however, some slow preflight readjustment to your destination's schedule might ensure an alert first few travel days.

SHIFT WORK

About a quarter of American workers have schedules that differ from the usual nine to five. Steady evening hours seem to cause few sleep problems. Some people prefer steady night hours, for example, 11:00 P.M. to 7:00 A.M. These people tend to be short sleepers who can get by with unsteady sleep hours. They get work out of the way at night so that they can enjoy the whole day. Some night workers, however, are not as alert or as organized as they think. One air force researcher who arranged interviews with night workers found that most of them came late to the interview. Night workers often sleep fewer hours than they need to function optimally.

The most troublesome work schedule is the rotating shift, in which workers must cycle continually among day, evening, and night shifts. The more frequently the shift changes, the less tolerable it will be to the workers. If the shift changes to later hours, which is like the traveler flying westward with the sun, the change will be tolerated better than if the shift changes to an earlier hour. But employers and military staff designing work hours do not always take biological clocks into account, despite the obvious advantages.

Some people do seem to tolerate shift work better than others. Of course, people who do not like schedule shifts are less likely to take these jobs, but some people are forced to accept difficult work schedules that create a sometimes painful conflict between human biology and the industrial culture.

You can do only what your body can tolerate. If you sleep poorly because of your work schedule, you will probably have to change the schedule somehow—or endure it. If you are on steady night shifts, try to find steady sleep hours you can live with seven days a week. If you are on rotating shifts, try to change shifts less often but always toward a later rather than an earlier shift. As we get older, we are less able to tolerate shift changes and some people must reconcile their schedules to that fact.

But you need not be a long-distance traveler or shift worker to suffer trouble from a mistimed sleep clock. The following case shows how everyday sleep disorders can result from normal scheduling problems and demonstrates the importance of making adjustments gradually.

SLEEP DISORDERS FROM LATE RISING

A sleep-clock problem beset Ms. M., a patient at the sleep clinic. A woman in her thirties, she was accustomed to retiring at 2:00 A.M. and arising about 9:30 A.M. But she knew that starting in September, several months away, she would have to get up well before nine to take her young twins to kindergarten, and she dreaded the prospect of rising that early. She felt she could not function if anything forced her to get up before nine, and she had no idea how she was going to dress, feed, and send the children off to school under those circumstances. Ms. M. had tremendous willpower. She had managed to give up her consumption of things that might interfere with her normal sleep patterns, including coffee and tobacco. But still she was unable to get the sound sleep she needed.

For a few weeks, she forced herself to go to bed several hours earlier than usual, hoping she could fall asleep quickly and awaken well before nine the next morning. But her tactic did not work. She lay sleepless until about 2:00 A.M., her usual bedtime. Only then did she become drowsy enough to sleep.

Ms. M. thought she had tried every possible option. "What should I do?" she asked. The answer was, in fact, to go to bed earlier, only at a slower pace. Ms. M. had been on the right track when she started to retire earlier than usual, but she failed to realize that it takes time to readjust the sleep cycle. No one can simply alter the sleep schedule by hours and make the change overnight by sheer force of will. The only way to do it is to accustom the body gradually to the desired schedule of sleep.

That is what Ms. M. ultimately did. At first she took the small step of always getting out of bed a half-hour before normal, at 9:00 A.M. Her bedtimes did not move commensurately earlier at first, thus contracting her sleep times and causing fatigue. Shorter periods of time in bed do, however, produce more solid sleep (see chap. 11). Furthermore, despite body clocks, fatigue eventually gets a person to sleep if a regular and progressive routine, such as Ms. M.'s, is followed. It took her a few weeks to settle into her new schedule. But she still had trouble getting up before nine. Fortunately, there were still some months left before her twins started kindergarten, so she and her doctor drew up a sleep schedule that got her out of bed five minutes earlier every other morning. Thus, she would be able to move her wake-up time back from 9:00 to 7:00 A.M. in about seven weeks. Before long, her bedtimes moved earlier and she was retiring regularly at 11:45 P.M.

Then a problem arose. Ms. M. took a night course that let out at 10:30 P.M. That left her insufficient time to relax and go to bed by the desired hour. To adjust, she compromised and went to bed at 11:30 on her free nights. On her class nights she retired a little later. This was not quite the desired schedule, but it worked. She started waking up at a time she had previously thought unthinkable: 7:30 A.M. By the time her children started kindergarten, Ms. M. was in bed by 11:45 each night and awoke at 7:30 the following morning. She got the children ready for school and on their way with no difficulty.

Ms. M. also felt much better, not only because she was relieved at being able to fulfill her morning's obligations but because late sleeping itself can make a person feel worse (see chap. 7). Years ago a California psychiatrist, George Globus, described a late-sleeping syndrome in which people feel out of sorts when they sleep late in the morning. Some people even feel fine when they first awaken, for example at 6:00 A.M., but then feel groggy and depressed if they return to sleep and arise at 9:00 A.M. More recently, researchers at the National Institutes of Health (NIH) demonstrated that making certain depressed people arise earlier improves their mood. Apparently a regular early rising time helps your attitude, and it also helps you meet your social obligations.

Ms. M. knew she had a problem with her internal clock, but not everyone who has a problem realizes it. Some insomnia patients think they maintain a regular sleep/wake schedule. When they keep a month's record of their actual bedtimes and hours of arising, however, they are surprised to see great irregularities. Figure 4 shows the irregular arising times of a 25-year-old data processor. He shows the common pattern of staying up late weekends on days 5 and 6, 12 and 13. On day 18 he starts a vacation and stays up increasingly late during the vacation. On day 21 he goes to bed early so he can resume his work schedule the next morning. But sleep schedules cannot be moved earlier in large jumps, and he lies awake for $2^1/_2$ hours after he goes to bed.

In figure 5, another patient shows a pattern of irregular arising times between 6:00 and 8:30 A.M. Many people can do this, but not someone who has chronic insomnia at night. Note that on many days the patient lies awake for more than two hours before falling asleep. A regular arising time lets the body know how many hours to spend awake and also when to sleep, but this patient is not giving her body the correct signals. The lengthy periods awake, both after bedtime and before arising, also indicate that this person is lying in bed too long.

The importance of a regular sleep schedule does not mean you should live with one eye on a stopwatch, regulating your sleep according to a rigid timetable. Your waking life will not suffer if you go to bed a couple of hours late every now and then. Indeed, an occasional deviation from a regular baseline will not greatly change your circadian rhythms. Everyone has to allow for the vagaries of work, family life, school, and social

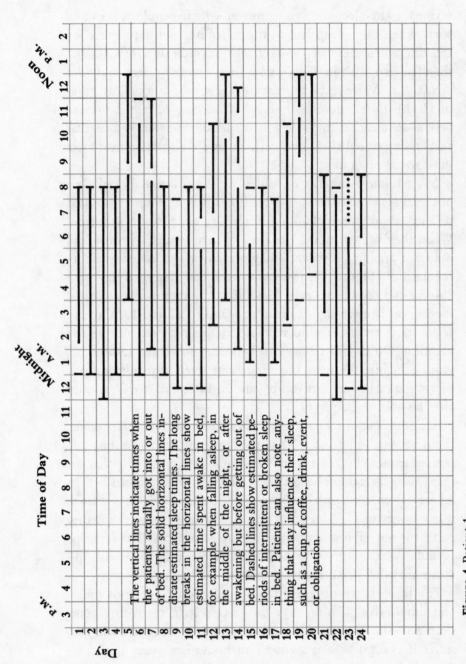

The vertical lines indicate times when the patients actually got into or out of bed. The solid horizontal lines indicate estimated sleep times. The long breaks in the horizontal lines show estimated time spent awake in bed, for example when falling asleep, in the middle of the night, or after awakening but before getting out of bed. Dashed lines show estimated periods of intermittent or broken sleep in bed. Patients can also note anything that may influence their sleep, such as a cup of coffee, drink, event, or obligation.

Figure 4 Patient 1.

The sleep charts of two insomnia patients show irregularities in the patients' bedtimes and arising times over the course of a month.

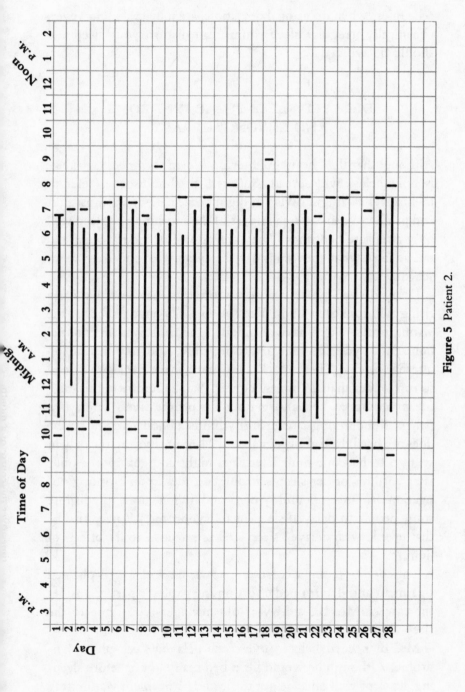

Figure 5 Patient 2.

schedules, when occasional deviations are inevitable. However, chronically irregular sleep timing can disturb your sleep and should be avoided.

DELAYED SLEEP-PHASE SYNDROME
AND CHRONOTHERAPY

Although hardly a household term, *delayed sleep-phase syndrome* is nonetheless widespread. Sufferers of this disorder refer to themselves as "night owls" or night people. They are most alert and productive in the small hours of the morning and sleep well only after late bedtimes. They get up late in the morning and rail against what they consider the tyranny of morning work schedules.

Delayed sleep-phase syndrome sufferers may fear that early rising will ruin their lives. They sleep easily enough, but at the wrong times. They have abandoned the timing of an external light/dark cycle, or regular arising time, and rely instead on internal clocks. These clocks, however, have cycles that tend to run longer than 24 hours. Longer than 24 hours, in this case, means going to bed and getting up progressively later. If a patient's underlying circadian rhythm is 25 hours and he or she does not heed the timing signals of a 24-hour rhythm, the patient will go to bed one hour later each night and get up one hour later until his or her sleep schedule intrudes upon morning obligations. (Thus unemployment and living alone predispose some people to delayed sleep-phase syndrome.) It may also be that people with delayed sleep are less sensitive to the effects of light.

The condition can be corrected, however, with a well-planned treatment and determined effort on the patient's part. Consider the case of Mr. B., a 34-year-old manager who came to the sleep clinic for help with his insomnia.

Mr. B. needed help to overcome delayed sleep-phase syndrome. Although he would lie in bed many hours before sleeping, he slept well once he got to sleep. His problem was getting to sleep and waking up early enough the following morning.

When time came to get up, he continued sleeping. He was free to sleep late on weekends and holidays if he wished, but he had no such freedom on weekdays, when, in order to go to work, he would get out of bed at an early hour feeling disoriented, depressed, and lethargic. When he did arise later, he felt much better, except that the late rising would delay his next night's sleep even longer. If he gave in to this delaying tendency, he would soon find himself awake all night and asleep all day.

This is the dilemma of the delayed sleep-phase syndrome patient: sleep well and be out of step with the rest of the world, or suffer by getting up when everyone else does. Such people have abandoned the 24-hour schedule in favor of a slightly longer schedule, and waking hours begin moving steadily later into the day until a conflict arises with morning work obligations. At this point the progression toward ever-later hours must cease, as it did in Mr. B.'s case. He would get up at the last possible moment, go to bed late, sleep late on weekends, and feel terrible much of the time. Mr. B.'s malaise probably resulted because the timing of his sleep-wake cycle no longer coincided with the timing of one or more of his other physiological systems. Irregular rising times further worsened his sleep, and sleeping late made him feel worse, an effect of Globus late-sleeping syndrome (see p. 52). Mr. B. always felt caught between his sleep inclinations and his work hours.

The underlying tendency toward later bedtimes often emerges as soon as a person escapes from the influence of daily pacemakers, such as regular office hours. Figure 6 tracks the sleeping schedule of a patient whose vacation began on day 18. Sleep times on successive nights got steadily later so that on day 25, for example, she did not arise until 10:30 A.M. Clearly, this patient needed regular work hours to keep her on a regular schedule.

Figure 7 shows an extreme example of delayed sleep-phase syndrome. This is the chart of a 34-year-old graduate student who had to attend a morning meeting one or two days a week, but otherwise had no fixed work schedule. After the five-to-six-day episodes of progressive delays in his bedtime, he attempted to get to sleep earlier and sometimes succeeded, as on

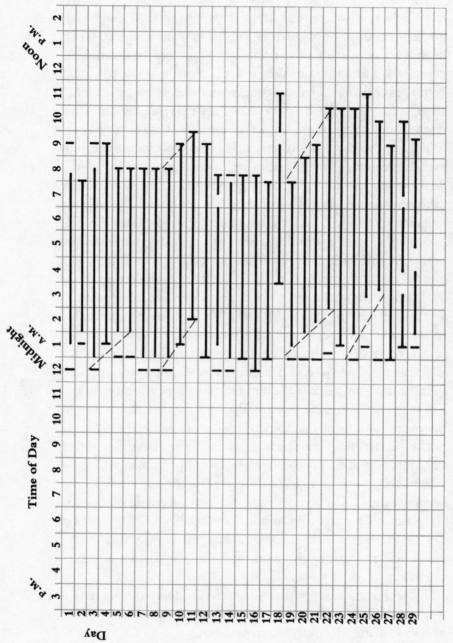

Figure 6 Successively later sleep times in an insomnia patient after starting vacation.

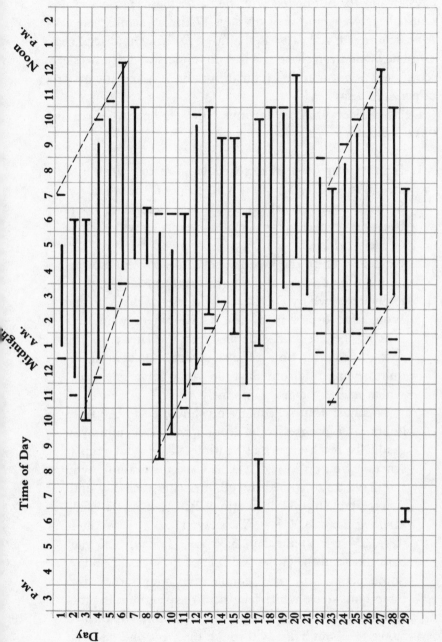

Figure 7 Sleep chart of an insomnia patient who had a fixed work schedule only two days a week.

days 15 and 16. But he felt wretched after these episodes, as his unusual early-evening naps on days 17 and 29 signify. He also felt discouraged, and castigated himself for being undisciplined. Until he made sleep charts, he had not understood that his sleep schedule was not merely irregular but also a systematic pattern of periodic delay.

Delayed sleep-phase syndrome can be relieved. There are three basic steps:

1. Fix a regular sleep/wake schedule no matter when it is, 2:30 A.M. to 10:30 A.M., 4 A.M. to noon, or whatever. Some patients are ashamed to reveal their sleep hours because they feel so abnormally out of step with the rest of the world.

2. Gradually shift the regular schedule toward normal hours. One method of doing this is *chronotherapy,* originally described by Dr. Charles Czeisler of Brigham and Women's Hospital in Boston. Chronotherapy involves moving the sleep schedule progressively later until you reach a desirable time. The sleep schedule shifting requires being off from daytime work for a full week, which makes the program costly.

   To adjust your schedule, you should go to bed three hours later progressively around the clock until you gradually reach a normal bedtime. If on your regular schedule you go to bed at 2:30 A.M., for example, you will have to go to bed three hours later each day until you reestablish an 11:30 bedtime: 2:30 A.M. Sunday, 5:30 A.M. Monday, 8:30 A.M. Tuesday, 11:30 A.M. Wednesday, 2:30 P.M. Thursday, 5:30 P.M. Friday, 8:30 P.M. Saturday, and the target bedtime of 11:30 P.M. Sunday. Some people can only handle two-hour rather than three-hour steps, which lengthens the program. In practice, however, some people shift bedtime forward to 5:00 P.M. about halfway through the week and find that they can get to sleep before midnight on subsequent nights.

3. When you've corrected delayed sleep-phase syndrome

and established a regular sleep-wake schedule for normal, desirable hours, the third and all-important step is to maintain the hours, thus preventing a relapse. The same problems that cause the delayed sleep-phase syndrome in the first place may still be there. There might be lessened sensitivity to the effects of light, a lack of equilibrium between the body's two clocks, or a feeling of wakefulness around normal bedtime. Once good hours have been reestablished, you must implement the masterstroke of schedule maintenance: Get up every morning at the same clock time, seven days a week, all the time. As soon as delayed sleep-phase syndrome patients give in a little—sleeping late on weekends or holidays—they ratchet their schedule forward, to a later hour, and find themselves increasingly awake at night. Then they must repeat the whole chronotherapy routine over again.

Trouble lurks when daylight savings time changes the clock time one hour earlier in the fall. For the delayed sleep-phase patient who has established a regular arising time, getting up an hour earlier usually proves possible. Jet travel eastward, of course, moves the schedule earlier, directly opposing the later-moving tendency of the clocks. Usually, however, the delayed sleep-phase patient who has a solidly predictable sleep-wake schedule can make the necessary adjustments, so long as the patient observes a steady arising time, no matter where he or she is.

Chronotherapy is also effective for those people who suffer from the opposite problem, *advanced* sleep-phase syndrome, in which they go to bed earlier and earlier and eventually are unable to stay awake past early evening. They sleep well, but cannot sleep beyond about 3:00 A.M. This syndrome occurs often in people over 65, because later in life our internal circadian rhythms shorten to a less-than-24-hour cycle and sleep comes earlier (see chap. 8). One older patient from Florida reported to her doctor that her friends were displeased if their dinner invitations were for anytime after 6:00 P.M., and that night life among the retired community ended around 9:00 P.M. To deal with advanced sleep-phase syndrome, the patient should adopt the same tactic used for delayed sleep-phase, but in reverse: arise progressively earlier each day.

There are other approaches to chronotherapy, although they all have the same basic goal of reforming the schedule. A more gradual chronotherapy technique is to move back your rising time 10 minutes every other day, but only after establishing a very regular rising time. This is what Ms. M. did before her twins entered kindergarten. It takes longer to show results, but does not require you to take a week off from work or otherwise upset your daily routine greatly.

Phase-response chronotherapy is also used to treat sleep-phase syndromes. If a patient stays wide awake in bright light for a timed 15-minute period just after the midpoint of a night's sleep, the exposure to simulated daylight (staring at a light bulb, reading with a bright light at book level, or using a bank of fluorescent lights) will send a signal to the internal sleep clock and shift the time the patient becomes sleepy in the evening. It is crucial to time the simulated daylight exactly. Exposure to the light before the midpoint can have just the opposite effect from the one desired. This means a patient must first establish a very regular sleep schedule. To get to sleep earlier, sessions in artificial light are scheduled after the midpoint of a patient's night. Assuming the patient has no sleep problem besides delayed sleep-phase syndrome, he or she will probably get back to sleep afterward and awaken at the usual time. That night, the patient goes to bed 15 or 20 minutes before the established bedtime, and the method is repeated until he or she is back to the desired sleep schedule.

Human biological design is not perfect. Some of our problems result when we must adjust our biological survival mechanisms to norms of behavior expected in a civilized society. Thus we suffer the scheduling problems of those who abandon the sun for electric light and who undertake long journeys with the aid of jet travel. The friction between our physiological timing systems, or internal clocks, and the external array of artificial schedules inevitably confuses the daily rhythms of life. We have seen how the timing of the sleep-wake cycle is thrown off by changes in light and modifications in our daily habits. Our internal clocks, related to basic life processes, can change only gradually. The treatment of biological clock disturbances, therefore, also requires slow and persistent adjustments. Unfortunately, some people might seek quick results themselves and force schedule changes that conflict with internal clocks. These people will inevitably suffer poor sleep and lessened alertness.

4

....

Caffeine

"The government of a nation is often decided over a cup of coffee," said historian G. P. R. James. One might say the same about a night's sleep. Caffeine is everywhere; about 80 percent of adults in the United States use it. Like other stimulants, caffeine reduces sleep quality. People who sleep poorly should avoid it completely.

Caffeine slips into your diet through several sources, from colas to candy bars. Table 1 lists a few selected foods and their approximate caffeine content. Caffeine is not necessarily confined to food and drink: some over-the-counter pain remedies and diet pills contain this stimulant. The caffeine content of the pills varies and can be anywhere from about 30 to 100 milligrams per tablet. Thus some people consume a gram or more of caffeine per day (a gram is about the weight of a small paper clip), although most ingest less than the amount contained in four cups of coffee. The amount of caffeine in a cup of tea or in two or three colas can keep the nerves of people who are sensitive to the substance on edge long afterward.

Food or drink	Caffeine content
Brewed coffee	80–170 mg per 6-oz. cup
Instant coffee	66–120 mg per 6-oz. cup
Leaf tea	30–90 mg per 6-oz. cup
Bag tea	42–100 mg per 6-oz. cup
Instant tea	30–60 mg per 6-oz. cup
Cocoa	Up to 50 mg per 6-oz. cup
Cola beverages	15–40 mg per 8-oz. glass
Chocolate bar	25 mg per 6-oz. bar
Chocolate cake	15 mg per slice

Caffeine could therefore take some of the blame for our seemingly sleepless society. Coffee and tea, the two most popular sources of caffeine, have much social and ceremonial importance. They are the focus of rituals from kaffeeklatsches to coffee breaks to tea ceremonies.

How people first began the caffeine habit is unknown. Tea has probably been drunk since prehistoric times, but tea plant cultivation began in China around the fourth century A.D. Venetian traders introduced Europe to tea in the late 1400s. It became a very popular drink, particularly with the British. Coffee beans were first made into a hot beverage in Ethiopia around 1000 A.D. Coffee drinking soon spread throughout the Arab world and was introduced to Europeans in the late 1500s. By the late 1600s, coffeehouses were extremely popular in Europe. Coffee was used in the American colonies as early as the 1600s, but became popular only after the British imposed a tea tax on the colonies. The resulting protests, one of which was the Boston Tea Party, restricted the colonists' tea supplies.

Any habit that has remained so popular for so long must have benefits. Of course, coffee and tea can be comforting. In addition to their pleasing taste and aroma, they warm the body and perk up the senses. A cup of coffee or tea can make a person feel more alert and stronger and even smarter for a while. But everything and everybody who goes up must come down, and caffeine definitely has its negative side. For one thing, it can trap the user in a vicious circle of sleep deprivation and overstimulation.

Caffeine continues to stimulate the user for 12 to 20 hours after it is consumed. This surprising result emerged from a study organized by the Coca-Cola Company in 1912. The manufacturers undertook research to see whether they should remove caffeine as an ingredient of Coca-Cola—just as they had previously removed cocaine. In the tests, the psychologist in charge could tell at 9:00 A.M. whether a volunteer had taken a dose of caffeine at 1:00 P.M. the previous afternoon. It was eventually decided that caffeine was benign enough to leave in Coca-Cola. Still, the duration of caffeine's effect means that after it gets you started in the morning it can still interfere with sound, refreshing sleep that night. Late at night, after the sleeper has been without caffeine for many hours, caffeine presents its down side. Still in the down, or withdrawal, period at his or her normal arising time, a caffeine user wakes up feeling groggy and thinks, "What I need is a cup of coffee to wake me up." Questionnaire surveys have revealed that people who use caffeine are actually groggier on first awakening than others who avoid caffeine.

Thus, a cycle is established. The morning cup of coffee keeps users stimulated for another long period, wrecks the sleep quality of some, and the cycle ends with drug-withdrawal grogginess the next morning. The cycle keeps repeating itself as long as your morning starts with coffee or tea.

In pure form, caffeine is a bitter-tasting white powder, one of a large family of drugs known as *alkaloids*. These nitrogen-bearing compounds are derived from plants, and some of them act on the nervous system and affect the mind. Several alkaloids have sinister reputations. Cocaine, an alkaloid derived from the coca plant, is one of the most addictive substances known. Strychnine, another alkaloid, is used for rat poison. Atropine, another poison, is found in deadly nightshade and has a powerful influence on actions of the brain, gut, bladder, eyes, glands, lungs, and heart.

The caffeine molecule resembles that of *adenosine,* a substance naturally present in the nervous system that acts to prevent neurotransmitter release. Nerve cells must fire at exactly the right time because nerve-cell circuitry bears information and controls and oversees the body's responses. Adenosine helps stabilize the system against unwanted nerve-cell firing. Caffeine, with its similar structure, can occupy some of the receptor sites on the surface of the nerve cell that would ordinarily be occupied by adenosine. Thus it lessens some of adenosine's inhibiting effects on nerve-cell firing—in other words, caffeine makes neurotransmission or nerve-cell firing easier.

Caffeine may not be as harmful, gram for gram, as cocaine or strychnine, but regular use of it may aggravate heart-rhythm disturbances, stomach problems, anxiety, and breast disease. (The breast is tissue modified from sweat glands, and caffeine's stimulation of the skin probably entails stimulation of the breasts as well. Inflammation of breast tissues can thus be worsened.) Surveys have shown that those who use larger amounts of caffeine also are likely to use more nicotine and more minor tranquilizers. In other words, heavy caffeine use may indicate a drug-taking tendency.

Other surveys have asked hospitalized patients to list symptoms they attribute to caffeine use. Here are some of the symptoms, with the most common ones first: frequent urination, insomnia, headaches from withdrawal of caffeine, diarrhea, anxiety, rapid heartbeat, tremulousness, and abdominal pain. Abdominal pain may arise either from the irritating effect coffee and tea have on the stomach or from the stimulating effect caffeine has on the bowels.

In patients who have panic attacks or fears that make it difficult for them to leave their homes *(agoraphobia),* researchers have found that caffeine increases nervousness, fear, nausea, restlessness, and other such disturbing symptoms in them to a much greater degree than in other people. A laboratory test involving the secretion of a stress-stimulated hormone, *cortisol,* is used to determine if a person is suffering from physically unhealthy levels of stress. In some cases, caffeine can make that test read positive.

There are worse drugs than caffeine, of course. The same surveys that show the harmful effects of nicotine use and alcohol abuse also indicate that low or moderate use of caffeine poses little hazard to a healthy individual. But caffeine can worsen a few preexisting problems such as peptic ulcers, cystic breast

disease, and heart disturbances. And even though caffeine, unlike nicotine or alcohol, will spare your lungs and liver, it certainly disrupts sleep.

EXCESSIVE SLEEPINESS CAUSED BY CAFFEINE

Caffeine not only can keep you awake, but also, under some
circumstances, can make you drowsy when you cannot afford
to be, and sometimes it even puts you to sleep. How does
caffeine, a stimulant, bring on sleepiness? The answer again
relates to the saying "What goes up must come down."

Adenosine assists you in certain tasks where you must adjust
your arousal level. Such tasks include coping with pain, choosing which features in your field of vision are worth reacting to,
and deciding which clues are important in a problem you must
solve. When adenosine is inhibited by caffeine, the nerve cells
fire more easily. Thus, caffeine opens up more sites in nerve
endings where the neurotransmitters are stored. Neurotransmitters such as norepinephrine and dopamine signal other nerve
cells when to fire, and so caffeine makes for more nerve-cell
firing in general.

Yet caffeine does not cause more of the neurotransmitters to
be produced. Before long, the supply of neurotransmitters runs
down and must be replenished. You feel stimulated in the first
hours after consuming caffeine because you are using more
neurotransmitters. Afterward, however, when neurotransmitter depletion catches up with you, you feel sluggish and drowsy,
and you must spend some time restoring your supply.

Thus, the effect of caffeine on the nervous system resembles
that of drugs like *amphetamine,* or "speed." It is also why the
"speed freak"—or even the heavy caffeine user—cannot regain
his or her initial "high" after "crashing" (that is, using up his
or her store of neurotransmitters). The price the stimulant user
pays for the period of stimulation is a subsequent prolonged
period of weakness and sluggishness.

This explanation, however, can only suggest what happens
in an individual caffeine user. Caffeine may affect some people

much more than others, because everyone has his or her own individual profile of various types of nerve cells that are sensitive to certain neurotransmitters. Thus some people are affected by caffeine far more than others. Some people remain perpetually sleepy beneath episodes of caffeine stimulation, despite the lengthy action of the drug. Possible explanations might be that the actions of caffeine diminish with continual use, or that caffeine has other actions in some people besides its well-known stimulation effect.

Whatever the explanation, regular caffeine use leaves people feeling generally groggier in the morning before they have a cup of coffee. Withdrawal from caffeine, when one must pay the penalty for exhausting too much of the neurotransmitter supply, can bring on weeks or months of sleepiness. The following case histories demonstrate this effect.

APPARENT NARCOLEPSY CAUSED BY CAFFEINE

To the casual observer, Ms. R. acted like a person with narcolepsy. After she began working in an office full-time, she began having 5- to 30-minute episodes during which she could hardly keep her eyes open; about 2:00 P.M. was her worst time. The afternoon attacks of sleepiness did not incapacitate Ms. R. completely. She stayed awake during them, and could remember afterward what had happened. She was able to answer phone calls, operate a copy machine, and perform other simple, repetitive tasks. But any work that called for alertness and initiative was beyond her during these attacks.

Ms. R. also had great trouble arising from bed in the morning, unlike people with narcolepsy, for whom early mornings are the most wakeful times. Laboratory recordings of her sleep had revealed no signs of narcolepsy. On one occasion, however, Ms. R. had been diagnosed as having the disorder. She had been placed temporarily on a stimulant medication, which had made her nervous. Ms. R. had no history or signs of narcolepsy, such as sudden muscle weakness or bad dreams, nor had she ever shown depressive symptoms. Tests for any underlying physiological causes revealed nothing of substance. All this deepened the mystery of her sleepiness.

Ultimately, the reason for Ms. R.'s problem was arrived at by process of elimination, and caffeine was found to be the source of her sleep troubles. Ms. R.'s daily caffeine intake was impressive. She consumed six to seven cups of coffee every day, plus an occasional cola drink. That added up to more than half a gram of caffeine daily. Her doctors had thought she used caffeine because she was sleepy, not the other way around. But her difficulty getting out of bed in the morning was typical of heavy caffeine users and so was her sleepiness around 2:00 P.M.

Ms. R. was advised to withdraw gradually, over several weeks, from using caffeine. She was also advised to take naps on weekend afternoons as needed. Ms. R. kept a written record of her progress over a four-week period. At first her record showed that caffeine withdrawal caused headaches and made her *more* drowsy, a very practical observation.

Many people, especially those who use caffeine heavily, find themselves so groggy and slow when they quit caffeine that they end up deciding caffeine is something they can't do without. People have been slowed down and even depressed for weeks—or months—after they quit. Unfortunately, they do not realize that caffeine withdrawal symptoms can last so long, and they mistakenly resume using caffeine rather than waiting for withdrawal symptoms to end.

After Ms. R. quit using caffeine, the sleepy periods gradually became fewer and shorter, and she began recording one "very good" day after another. In time, her "narcoleptic" sleepiness was totally relieved by abstinence from caffeine. Ms. R.'s problem is more common than most people think.

CAFFEINE WITHDRAWAL: A COMMON PROBLEM

Ms. B. provides another example of how caffeine can actually cause sleepiness. She was a nurse who had always struggled to wake up in the morning. As a child, she took an hour to awaken fully, and sometimes she would nod off at the breakfast table. As an adult, she frequently felt sleepy and lethargic during the day. Sometimes, on her day off, she would sleep 16 hours. Ms. B. actually had none of the clear signs of narcolepsy, such as brief, daily naps. On the whole, she seemed to be in good health; nothing in her daily experience seemed unusual for a nurse.

Ms. B.'s troubles centered on her 10-cup-a-day coffee habit. This became apparent when she was required to stop drinking coffee so that it would not disturb results of laboratory investigations of her sleepiness. Ms. B. quit "cold turkey" while on a vacation. She felt better almost immediately. In her caffeine-free condition she no longer felt lethargic and found she could function adequately on as little as four hours' sleep a night. Suddenly she needed no further treatment. But she still wanted a hot beverage from time to time, so she substituted caffeine-free herbal tea for coffee. Ms. B. was more fortunate than most caffeine users because she did not have uncomfortable withdrawal symptoms such as headaches and grogginess.

Ms. R.'s and Ms. B.'s episodes of drowsiness would seem to contradict our usual notions about caffeine: the drug is supposed to stimulate, not sedate. Caffeine users interpret any sedated mood that follows their "high" as a need for more caffeine. After a while, the draggy feeling that accompanies the erosion of one's neurotransmitter stores begins to feel like a normal state rather than a drug-induced low. But this low can have significant effects on behavior and health, as illustrated in Mr. N.'s case.

It took a near-fatal accident to motivate Mr. N. to seek treatment for his sleep disorder. A young man who frequently felt sleepy during the day, Mr. N. had been involved in two serious automobile accidents in the evening after work. In one of them, his car swerved into oncoming traffic and was hit by a truck. The accident fractured his jaw, cut his nose badly, and caused major injuries to his hand. In addition, he faced legal trouble: a "driving to endanger" citation stood to deprive him of his driver's license, which he needed in his work. Since Mr. N.'s accident happened to him when he was driving home in the evening, the plastic surgeon who repaired his face and hand suspected a sleep disorder might be responsible and referred him to a sleep clinic.

It turned out that Mr. N. had some other problems. He slept late on weekend mornings, often another sign of excessive sleepiness. His nose was frequently stuffed. He snored loudly, and his heavy smoking had impaired his lung function. All this indicated he might have sleep apnea (see chap. 10), which can make a person very drowsy. Furthermore, his father, who also snored heavily, had died in an auto accident, probably after falling asleep at the wheel. This made Mr. N.'s doctors further suspect sleep apnea because there may be an hereditary factor to the disorder.

To check for sleep apnea, the doctors made a recording of Mr. N.'s night sleep in the sleep laboratory. Mr. N. fell asleep within three minutes and had more REM sleep and more body movements than expected. But none of the laboratory information clearly accounted for his sleepiness. In particular, he showed no signs of sleep apnea.

With no firm diagnosis, the trail of clues led once more to drug use. Mr. N. drank four or five cups of coffee each day and about a quart of cola drinks, taking in perhaps 600 milligrams of caffeine daily. Withdrawal each evening from that much caffeine might account for Mr. N.'s sleepiness, or perhaps the excess stimulation from caffeine during the day might have hurt the quality of Mr. N.'s sleep, as indicated by the increased REM and body movements found in the laboratory. Mr. N.'s nicotine habit might also help to keep him up nights.

Mr. N.'s therapy consisted of three parts. He got off caffeine, gave up smoking, and established a regular sleep/wake schedule with regular arising times on weekends as well. Before long he was back to a normal, active workday routine and had no more drowsiness when driving. Because his treatment at the sleep clinic revealed that his accidents were probably due to stimulant use and not to irresponsibility, he was allowed to keep his driver's license.

A year and a half later, his doctor telephoned Mr. N. to see how he was doing. He still drove in the evenings without feeling sleepy, and he still got up at regular times each day, including weekends. He remained off caffeine but was back on cigarettes, half a pack a day—an indication of how addicting nicotine is.

Many people use caffeine to help themselves wake up. But the preceding examples show that it may cause sleepiness. Generally, severe cases of drowsiness like those just described accompany exceptionally heavy use of caffeine. They also usually involve a mistake. The person believes that he or she simply must be a sleepy person and needs caffeine to stay awake. The drowsiness one feels upon giving up the drug may last for weeks or even months. But after that much time the ex-coffee drinker discounts drug withdrawal as a plausible cause for his or her sleepiness and mistakenly assumes that a constant caffeine habit is the remedy rather than the cause of his or her problem.

Caffeine may cause sleepiness in some cases simply by lessening sleep. Figure 8 shows the sleep chart of a 30-year-old internist who drank two to four cups of coffee and a cup of tea or two daily. The chart shows she was on call many nights and had plenty of wakeful periods in the midst of her sleep. She complained of great fatigue in the morning and had trouble concentrating during morning conferences.

Figure 9 shows her off all caffeine and keeping a regular arising time of 7:00 A.M., regardless of bedtime. This month she had to work on call more often than the first month. Despite this, she averaged more sleep per night the second month than the first, about 6.2 hours per night compared with 5.2 hours. Thus the caffeine deprived her of more sleep than an increased nightwork schedule did. Notice that she slept worse when she had alcoholic drinks in the evening (see chap. 5).

CAFFEINE SENSITIVITY

More often than sleepiness, caffeine use brings on insomnia. A few years ago, charts of sleep-clinic patients revealed that people experiencing insomnia at the beginning of the night used much more caffeine than others, including those who awoke too early in the morning and those who had disturbed sleep the whole night long. This suggested that the stimulation of caffeine still

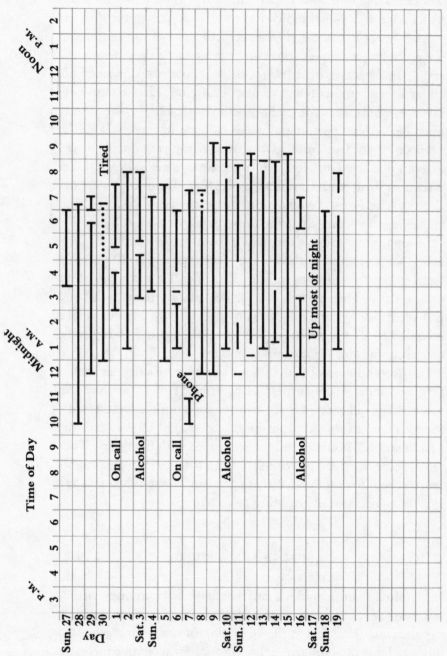

Figure 8 Thirty-year-old internist's sleep chart, first month, while using caffeine.

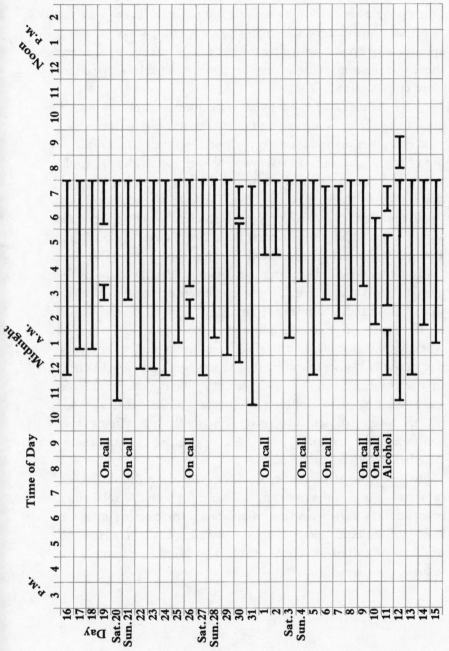

Figure 9 Thirty-year-old internist's sleep chart, second month, after discontinuing use of caffeine.

operated strongly enough at bedtime to keep the person awake. Some people are extremely sensitive to caffeine. There was, for example, an insurance salesman who was kept awake by a few spoonfuls of chocolate ice cream but not by raspberry sherbet; there was the housewife whose sleep was spoiled by three chocolate chip cookies.

Many people have relieved their insomnia simply by totally avoiding caffeine. One young laboratory technician in the hospital called her doctor for a sleep-clinic appointment, complaining of insomnia. She had always slept well, but suddenly could not, even though she said nothing had changed in her life. She drank two or three cups of coffee a day. Her doctor told her to discontinue it and to keep a sleep chart prior to her first appointment. She phoned back after a few days to cancel her appointment because good sleep had returned.

"But why would discontinuing coffee have relieved the problem," the doctor asked, "if you had been drinking coffee for years before the insomnia appeared?"

She explained that the laboratory coffeepot had stopped working and that she had begun drinking the coffee down the hall in the radiotherapy unit. It was stronger and tasted better. That was when her insomnia appeared. When the pot was fixed and she returned to drinking the more ordinary coffee in her lab, the sleep problem vanished. Apparently her caffeine dose had exceeded a certain level that was critical for her, and thereafter her sleep was disrupted.

Just one cup of coffee at breakfast can make the difference between a good and a poor night's sleep for some people, since everyone has varied degrees of tolerance for caffeine. But the legion of coffee drinkers who sleep well tends to obscure the problem of caffeine-caused insomnia in highly sensitive individuals.

5

....

Alcohol, Tobacco, and Medications

In Shakespeare's *Macbeth,* the porter summarizes the action of alcohol this way: "Beer, sir, is a great provoker of . . . sleep and urine." Shakespeare's words are true, up to a point. Drinking beer does stimulate the output of urine and induce a groggy condition that leads to sleep. (Indeed, the expression "groggy" is derived from grog, the shipboard rum drink rationed to British sailors during Britain's imperial days.) But alcohol does not encourage sound sleep. On the contrary, it interferes with uninterrupted sleep. So those with significant sleep problems who think "a little drink" (or two or three) before bedtime will help them sleep are likely to be disappointed.

This is not to say that the teetotaler is guaranteed refreshing sleep, nor that slumber is doomed by a sip of beer or wine. The moderate, sensible drinker probably sleeps no worse than anyone else. But heavy alcohol use, in an effort to bring on sleep, or even the habit of taking a nightcap before retiring, can harm sleep quality.

MYTHS AND REALITIES OF ALCOHOL

Alcohol is the universal drug, used and abused almost everywhere. It has many effects on organs and systems, including the brain. The blood-brain barrier, a physiological filter that prevents many harmful chemicals from reaching the brain, does not stop alcohol, which enters the brain and acts as a depressant and tranquilizer on the central nervous system. This effect is what makes alcohol soporific.

Alcohol also affects voluntary control of the body; it slows the sequencing and coordinating functions of the brain. Yet it is alcohol's effects on involuntary muscles that may interfere with sleep. For example, nerves leading to the muscles of the upper airway cause it to widen when a breath is taken so that air passes through easily. The airway widens less readily, however, after alcohol is consumed. This often causes the drinker to snore more loudly. Breathing may be so impaired that the sleeper must struggle to draw a breath, thus damaging sleep quality.

At the same time, alcohol, even though it sedates the user, may also increase levels of noradrenaline in the nervous system and keep them at relatively high levels for 12 hours or longer. In one study, noradrenaline remained at high levels for 14 hours. (Research data like this are often hard to obtain. To discover the effects of alcohol consumption on the nervous system, volunteers for the experiments must be willing to have a needle inserted in the lower spine to draw off a sample of cerebrospinal fluid for analysis.)

So, although alcohol may act first as a sedative and can help lull a person to sleep, it later disturbs sleep in several ways: by stimulating production of adrenalinelike neurotransmitters, by interfering with breathing in some people, and by increasing urine output, which awakens the sleeper with the urge to use the toilet. In sleep laboratory experiments, sleep is found to be generally worse after alcohol consumption.

Not everyone who drinks suffers the same degree of damage to sleep. It is difficult to predict exactly how alcohol will affect anyone's sleep, because individuals differ so greatly in their responses to it. A person can investigate how alcohol affects his or her sleep, however, by maintaining a sleep chart for a month or two and then evaluating how he or she slept, on the average, on nights when alcohol was consumed. The findings are then compared to nights when the person abstained (see chap. 11).

BREAKING THE GRIP OF ALCOHOL

Most patients seeking better sleep (or improved health in general) will discontinue drinking on the advice of a physician. It seems much easier for them to quit drinking than to stick to healthy eating habits or to quit nicotine. Most drinkers use alcohol moderately. Heavy drinkers are less able to quit, and their problems are well-known.

There is another type of drinker who uses alcohol moderately but steadily, yet apparently manages to function well. Such drinkers usually drink every evening and invariably their social occasions involve alcohol. They feel they can discontinue drinking easily at any time, but when advised to do so, they cannot. They deny that their drinking is a problem. Often they become very nervous if a hospital stay or other occasion forces them to give up drinking for a few days. It is often more difficult to convince moderate drinkers with insomnia to give up drinking, but many of them are surprised how much more soundly they sleep after quitting.

Alcoholics face more serious problems with sleep disorders. Years after the short-term effects of alcohol withdrawal are over, alcoholics may continue to suffer diminished sleep quality; their sleep is often lighter and more fragmented than normal. Only the alcoholic really understands what it means to overcome alcoholism. Nevertheless, the grip of alcoholism can be broken, as legions of sober alcoholics testify. Quitting is more likely if some form of treatment and group therapy is available to provide a sense of community support. This may be one reason for the success of Alcoholics Anonymous (AA), which has generally effective methods for relieving alcoholism and remains a component of most treatment facilities.

TOBACCO ADDICTION AND SLEEP DISORDERS

Of the many substances we take into our bodies, some, like caffeine, are likely to worsen people's sleep. Other substances, however, may not disturb everyone who uses them, but they can affect the sleep of some people a great deal. Tobacco belongs in this latter category. Experimental evidence indicates that smoking can interfere with sleep.

Quitting smoking is such a formidable challenge that an entire industry has arisen—marketing everything from books to nicotine chewing gum—solely to help the smoker break the tobacco habit. Even with such assistance tobacco addiction is hard to overcome. The insomnia sufferer who smokes faces perhaps the most difficult task of all patients afflicted by sleep disorders: giving up nicotine.

Yet cigarettes and other tobacco products must be given up to encourage sound, good-quality sleep. The more you smoke, the less you sleep, as revealed by an epidemiological survey carried out in England in 1980. Researchers there found that smoking one pack of cigarettes per day reduced sleeping by almost half an hour per night—a significant loss. In that same year Dr. Constantine Soldatos of the Hershey Medical Center in Pennsylvania, reported more encouraging results. He discovered that after only one week free from cigarettes, ex-smokers began sleeping better. They felt worse overall, of course, being in the throes of withdrawal, but they nevertheless slept more soundly.

Tobacco disrupts sleep in several ways. It contains nicotine, an alkaloid that in pure form is a faintly yellowish, oily liquid with a bitter taste, and is a powerful stimulant. Nicotine acts on the heart, blood vessels, nervous system, and many other organs. The nicotine content of tobacco varies from one strain to another; as a rule, low-grade tobacco is rich in nicotine, while higher grades, such as fine Turkish leaf, have less nicotine.

Nicotine has an exquisitely specific affinity for a type of cell in the autonomic nervous system that uses acetylcholine as its neurotransmitter. The autonomic nervous system controls the behavior of most internal organs. By taking acetylcholine's place in the nerve cells' receptor sites, nicotine increases the likelihood that the cell will fire, producing a variety of effects. A longtime smoker will respond differently to nicotine than a neophyte. Some people have more (or fewer) nerve cells that are affected by nicotine, and therefore will have a greater (or lesser) reaction. The heart may be slowed or quickened, depending on how much nicotine has been ingested, the time of day, and the user's physical makeup. Similarly, nicotine stimulates the adrenal gland, increasing adrenaline production, and constricts blood vessels, which raises blood pressure. Smokers seek the "rush" or "lift" associated with a release of adrenaline, but the intensity of the experience depends on the variables just mentioned. Nicotine also stimulates the gut, and acts upon many other organs, including the bladder, uterus, and salivary glands. Many structures of the central nervous system are also affected.

Although many of nicotine's ill effects account for the relatively poorer health of smokers, they do not explain the addictive power of the drug, which is greater than alcohol and similar to heroin. In one comparison study, for instance, about 80 percent of those quitting heroin or nicotine had relapsed within a year, compared with about 70 percent of alcoholics. The physiological mechanism for nicotine addiction is not precisely known; nicotine receptors do not seem to account for addiction.

Nevertheless, one piece of evidence suggests that noradrenaline, a neurotransmitter discussed earlier as regulating REM sleep, may be involved in the mechanism of nicotine craving. Clonidine, a drug that acts specifically on nerve cells that respond to noradrenaline, seems to lessen the craving of nicotine addicts in the immediate withdrawal period. These nerve cells seem to be the center of those chemical processes that underlie craving. Clonidine's effect on craving is more specific than the action of a sedative that calms the restlessness, tension, and irritability of withdrawal. Some of the cells that respond to noradrenaline also have receptor sites on their outer walls that are sensitive to the action of opiates. Therefore, other severe addictions probably also involve the action of noradrenaline-sensitive nerve cells.

It is difficult to say how many Americans suffer from sleep disorders related to smoking, but many patients who seek help from sleep clinics are smokers, and because nicotine can affect sleep quality, part of their therapy is to give up the habit altogether.

Many smokers who try to quit completely and abruptly are likely to undergo intense withdrawal symptoms, including edginess, irritability, and an inability to concentrate. Some will gain weight; stimulants such as nicotine suppress one's appetite so the removal of these stimulants increases it. Still, the major symptom that is experienced is a craving for nicotine. This craving seriously tests the resolve of the ex-smoker, and the agonies of withdrawal drive many smokers back to tobacco.

The variety of quitting programs available testifies that no single one of them works for most smokers. Everyone must find the personal program that makes him or her feel most comfortable. Equally important are the people in the smoker's life who will help, including friends, family members, and professionals.

Currently, the major method of smoking cessation is short-term therapy groups that use instruction, group support, and behavior modification—a structured program of rewards, stress management, and gradual withdrawal. There are also private, freestanding organizations whose business is smoking cessation. Hypnosis, an idea many smokers find appealing, only works in a small percentage of cases. A psychologist experienced in nicotine withdrawal can help put together an individualized behavior-therapy program.

Here are some things for the smoker to consider before quitting:

First, the smoker might decide whether he or she is a high- or low-intake person. The high-intake person smokes continually, all day long. He or she maintains a steady blood level of nicotine and avoids withdrawal symptoms because the supply is constantly replenished. The heavy smoker who cannot get through a movie without grabbing a few puffs in the lobby is the same one who may also awaken in the middle of the night craving a cigarette because the nocturnal level of blood nicotine has fallen intolerably. Yet the heavy smoker with insomnia, like most patients whose sleep disorders stem from drugs, rarely recognizes why he or she cannot sleep. It often comes as a shock to the smoker that cigarettes are part of his or her sleep problems.

Low-intake smokers are also found among the ranks of insomnia patients. They are often young women who consume only four or five cigarettes per day, all in the evening. (Some low-intake smokers consume even fewer cigarettes, four or five per week, or even less.) These low-intake smokers probably cannot be considered physiologically addicted, but they still have the potential to get hooked. They enjoy the rapid rush they get from the suddenly rising blood-nicotine level. The nicotine then is allowed to clear enough so that the next cigarette causes another pleasant stimulation.

After determining if he or she is a high- or low-intake smoker, the smoker must decide which way to give up smoking: gradually or cold turkey. Each approach has its benefits.

Gradually reducing tobacco consumption minimizes withdrawal symptoms, but the withdrawal period usually must be extended for months. The smoker must guard against self-delusion about nicotine dependency. At the opposite extreme, the cold turkey approach may work best for low-intake smokers, since they will suffer fewer effects from withdrawal. Some heavy smokers, however, unsure of their ability to resist nicotine, feel they must quit completely and abruptly or not at all. These smokers choose to suffer the pangs of sudden withdrawal rather than the uncertainty of gradual cessation. The cold turkey method is precarious for some because it usually provokes huge cravings for nicotine. But for others it involves less risk, averting a prolonged and painful period of self-restraint. However one does it, ceasing smoking is hard work.

If you are a smoker, here are some specific, gradual withdrawal methods in use:

1. Chart when and in what circumstances you smoke each cigarette. Charting your smoking is a way to measure addiction. This record keeps the problem on your mind,

which is enough to make some smokers quit charting rather than smoking. Rank the cigarettes from the least to the most important ones of the day. The most important ones tend to be the first cigarette of the morning (probably because blood-nicotine levels reach a low during the night) and cigarettes smoked after meals (possibly due to repeated association with a pleasantly sated feeling). The least important cigarettes are those you pick up without thinking about it, as when you automatically light a cigarette while you talk on the telephone.

2. Plan a withdrawal period. Decide how long your nicotine-withdrawal period will be, then give up cigarettes gradually, over 60 to 80 days, starting with the least important one of the day on the first day and progressing to the most important ones.

3. Announce your intentions to others. Tell everyone you know that you plan to quit smoking, and get some close friends to quit smoking as well. All of these steps create a supportive atmosphere that will encourage you to quit.

4. Make your nicotine intake less potent. The nicotine content in cigarettes varies from brand to brand, and you can tell the level of nicotine of your brand by looking at the nicotine dose written on the package. Pick a brand with slightly less nicotine than the one you now smoke, and switch brands each week or two, working your way down to relatively weak cigarettes that will be easier to give up.

5. Try nicotine gum. It replaces cigarettes completely and is available by prescription. The gum delivers nicotine to the bloodstream more slowly than cigarettes do, but has helped many smokers wean themselves from tobacco. Overuse of the gum may cause unpleasant symptoms such as headache and nausea, but by trial and error you and your physician can determine the proper dose. Each time you crave a cigarette, place a piece of gum in your mouth and chew it three or four times, then

remove it from your mouth and store it in wax paper. Thereafter, experiment to see how much you need to chew to relieve the craving for a cigarette. (*Do not* resume smoking while you are on the gum; rather, increase your dose of nicotine gum.) Also, a liquid nicotine solution is sometimes used as nose drops to reduce nicotine craving. All these methods basically aim to help you give up cigarettes fast and nicotine gradually, though you do run the risk of becoming addicted to the nicotine in gum or drops.

6. Once you decide on a plan for giving up smoking, arrange a way of monitoring your progress, and have a good friend or confidant you can talk to if your resolution wavers.

7. If the cost is not too prohibitive, use professional groups that help people to stop smoking. These organizations are widely available and even many large corporations maintain them for their employees. Many hospitals also sponsor them. Programs employ many of the aforementioned methods and also organize groups of mutually supportive smokers under the guidance of a leader whose job it is to know about giving up nicotine. Methods vary from one session of instruction and suggestion using varied techniques, to monthlong or six-week-long sessions. Single-session programs often allow you to return for reinforcement sessions free. Program costs vary from about $100 per single session to $250 to $300 for the monthlong sessions.

CARBOHYDRATE CONSUMPTION AND SLEEP DISORDERS

People seldom think of sweets as stimulants, since sugar is not a drug like caffeine or nicotine. Yet a piece of candy, for some people, seems to have much the same effect as a cup of coffee or a cigarette. Many drowsy patients at sleep clinics report that they eat a piece of candy to fight daytime sleepiness, or they even claim to get a lift from sweets. But the question of whether sweets really provide stimulation has no definitive answer.

The stimulating effect of carbohydrates has been little investigated, so any discussion of carbohydrates is not backed up by the detailed research available on caffeine, alcohol, or nicotine. Actually, research shows that eating a meal high in carbohydrates makes people sleep a few hours later the next morning. But we have conflicting information from patients' observations, and while it is difficult to obtain information that applies to everyone, we can record the effects of a carbohydrate-rich meal eaten a few hours prior to bedtime. In specific cases some other ingredient in sweets besides carbohydrates might cause stimulation, or the patient might simply be responding to suggestions that eating carbohydrates delivers quick energy.

In a sleep clinic, where people are always talking about how alert or how sleepy they are, there is a consistency to the stories about carbohydrate stimulation. Many a drowsy sleep-apnea patient pops one candy after another into his or her mouth to keep awake while driving. One narcolepsy patient carried out an experiment to see which foods would help her get through her factory work shift. She kept records of what she ate and made fine distinctions among the effects of the various foods. A peanut butter sandwich, which probably had about 30 grams of carbohydrate, did not keep her awake as well as a peanut-butter-and-jelly sandwich, which contained about 50 grams of carbohydrate. This kind of story makes one consider that carbohydrates may possibly interfere with sleep in some people. Many patients, though not all, feel their sleep improves after drastically decreasing carbohydrate intake. It is not established exactly how reducing carbohydrate intake helps these people, but it helps nonetheless. The effect appears to be short-term: Carbohydrates eaten at breakfast have little effect on sleep, but carbohydrates eaten at dinner may disrupt sleep greatly.

In addition to a possible stimulating effect, carbohydrates can increase appetite. When a person feels hungry and eats a meal made up largely of carbohydrates, his or her blood sugar fluctuates. Blood-sugar levels go up soon after eating and then fall soon after he or she secretes insulin and metabolizes the carbohydrates. Eating protein with the carbohydrates moderates these fluctuations to some extent. These swings in blood-sugar level affect appetite. On the downswing of blood-sugar levels, appetite picks up, and the cycle starts again. There are some people whose appetite is controlled largely by this mechanism. They eat a lot of snacks and may take few actual meals, preferring to consume small amounts of food every few hours. This continual snacking reduces the timing information that their bodies receive from regular mealtimes, and this may interfere with the bodily clock function that sets the sleep/wake cycle.

CARBOHYDRATE-RELATED SLEEP DISORDERS

Mr. M., a banker in his thirties, was under treatment at a sleep clinic for insomnia, and his treatment, which involved scheduling his bedtimes, taking antidepressant medication, and discontinuing caffeine, had generally worked well. He was sleeping better at night and feeling better during the day. Yet there was room for improvement in the quality of his sleep, because he kept awakening in the middle of the night.

During a discussion at the sleep clinic, Mr. M. mentioned that he felt thirsty during these nighttime waking episodes and kept a container of cold orange juice on his night table to sip. Here was a factor that had been overlooked. As he relieved his thirst, he was also consuming carbohydrate calories in the middle of the night. This was bound to affect his appetite and, through it, his body's internal clocks.

Further investigation revealed that orange juice was not the only carbohydrate-rich food Mr. M. had been consuming at night. Cake, cookies, and pastries of all kinds were part of his evening ritual. To correct this condition, Mr. M. was told to have most of his day's carbohydrates at breakfast, eat a low-carbohydrate lunch, and have a salad for dinner. In following this regimen for the most part, he ceased to awaken in the middle of the night.

Carbohydrate-related sleeping problems do not always involve sleeplessness, nor are they always easy to detect. Sometimes carbohydrates aggravate excessive sleepiness. Persistent discussion and investigation are the only methods that can uncover the cause of the trouble. Consider the case of Ms. G., an overweight woman in her forties who felt drowsy during the day. She also had trouble with headaches, forgetfulness, and nightmares, but it was her sleepiness that brought her to a sleep clinic. She was so sleepy that she could drive her car for only a few minutes before drowsiness overcame her.

She performed poorly on vigilance tests at the clinic. One such test, the Continuous Performance Test, requires a patient to pay close attention and react rapidly to a series of letters displayed at a rate of one per second. Ms. G. could barely press the button indicating when she saw a particular letter. The psychologist who administered the test thought Ms. G. might be having one half to one second lapses every one to two seconds, even though she remained seated upright and appeared alert.

Her drowsiness had begun at the time she moved from one house to another. She thought perhaps she was allergic to something at the new house and that the allergy was responsible for her difficulties. Certainly she had plenty of work to do at the house, from painting to wallpapering. In addition, she had to take care of her three young children. For quick energy, Ms. G. began to eat sweets such as brownies and candy bars. Her weight soared upward by 40 pounds and her sleepiness increased gradually about this same time.

Was this the cause of her sleep disorder? To try and shed more light on the condition, she underwent a glucose tolerance test. Ms. G. went to a laboratory one morning, drank a very sweet liquid, and waited for six hours while blood was drawn periodically and analyzed to determine blood-sugar levels. Normally, blood glucose rises rapidly in a half hour and returns to normal after two hours. Results of her test were normal; they were also misleading. In fact, the glucose tolerance test sometimes has little predictive value and diagnostic usefulness. In real life Ms. G. did not usually sit around waiting for a blood sample to be taken; she was performing hard work, which consumes glucose. To find out what was really going on in her bloodstream, she would have to test her blood-sugar levels herself at home during the course of the day.

Ms. G. did so, using a home test kit, and found a pattern very different from that measured in the laboratory. Her blood sugar before breakfast was abnormally low, about 40 milligrams of sugar per 100 milliliters of blood. (A normal reading would range approximately between 60 mg and 110 mg per 100 ml, depending on the laboratory.) Her blood-sugar levels consistently fell this low again two hours after meals, probably because the insulin she secreted in response to her sweet meals overshot the mark, causing glucose to be metabolized and cleared from the bloodstream until her blood-sugar level was unusually low. Thus, she was getting too much sugar in the bloodstream at some times and too little at others. Low-sugar levels coincided with the times she felt drowsy.

Ms. G. was placed on a low-carbohydrate diet, and she followed it faithfully. She began to live mainly on low-starch vegetables, meat, fish, and cheese. Within six weeks, she lost 31 pounds, and her symptoms all abated. She could drive long distances again and feel totally alert. Much of her weight loss appeared to be water, since she had lost weight very rapidly and the puffiness in her face disappeared. While some effect of the carbohydrates may have kept her tissues full of water, Ms. G.'s weight loss was a mystery that defies easy explanation. Perhaps she had eaten more salty foods, such as nuts and potato chips, than she realized before she changed her diet (salt causes water retention), or possibly she had some undiagnosed condition causing accumulation of excess fluid that lessens with weight loss.

These cases, and those in the previous two chapters, illustrate an important principle used in treating sleep disorders: Whenever there is an unexplained problem, correct all surrounding irregularities—disordered sleep schedules, unbalanced diet, or whatever else—and eventually the explanation and probably the solution will appear.

DRUGS AND THEIR EFFECT ON SLEEP

Many over-the-counter and prescription medications can harm sleep quality. Nonprescription medicines commonly contain caffeine or other drugs that interfere with sound sleep. For example, widely used nasal sprays have stimulant actions that can damage sleep quality. Even if a medication can cause sleeplessness or excessive somnolence, a person cannot tell beforehand whether it can cause him or her sleep problems, because we all vary so much in our responses to drugs.

Sleep problems caused by a nonprescription medication usually can be relieved by stopping the medicine. It may be impossible to quit prescription drugs that are needed for a medical problem. This poses a conflict between sleep and other aspects of health. In such cases, physician and patient can work together to find out the most advantageous use of the drug while minimizing its sleep-disrupting influence. In such a collaboration, the patient may keep a chart of his or her sleep and of the symptoms to be relieved by the drug. The physician may monitor any laboratory test results that indicate how the drug might be acting and examine the effects of the medication, the times it is taken, the dosages, and how the medication's effects are modified by any other drugs the patient has taken.

Tracking drug interactions can be difficult. Hundreds of new pharmaceuticals appear on the market each year, with applications ranging from pain relief to immunotherapy. Keeping track of all these new compounds, their uses and effects, is a profession in itself. Classifying drugs is also difficult. For example, diazepam (Valium), frequently prescribed to reduce anxiety, is often classified as a tranquilizer. Yet it is also used as an anesthetic, an anticonvulsant, or antispastic drug in the treatment of cerebral palsy. It is not uncommon for a single drug to fall into several different categories, depending on its effects and intended uses. Therefore, patient and doctor must pay close attention to how the drug is used.

PRESCRIPTION VERSUS
NONPRESCRIPTION DRUGS

Although there is considerable overlap between some prescription and nonprescription drugs (sometimes the only difference between a prescription and nonprescription medication is the dosage), prescription drugs tend to be stronger and more specific in their effects than nonprescription medications. Yet both kinds can harm sleep if the user is unaware of their sleep-robbing potential.

Nonprescription decongestants frequently contain drugs that have stimulating effects. One such example is pseudoephedrine, a drug that constricts engorged blood vessels in the nose. Doctors have observed that some patients who suffer from excessive sleepiness keep themselves awake with pseudoephedrine. Phenylpropanolamine is another stimulating drug found frequently in cold remedies. In many cases other drugs (including antihistamines) are present in the same pill partly to fight allergic effects and partly to counteract the stimulation. One problematic aspect of these combinations of stimulants and sedatives is that they do not affect everyone in the same way; some people are more sensitive to the stimulant part, whereas others are more affected by the sedative.

When such drugs shrink the size of small blood vessels running through the inner lining of the nose, the engorged lining is blanched and stops secreting excess mucus. But the vessel shrinking done by these nasal decongestants is due to their adrenalinelike actions. So when the drugs taken orally or inhaled to shrink swollen membranes are transported into the nervous system, their stimulating actions can disrupt sleep.

Stimulant medications found in over-the-counter nasal sprays are popular during allergy seasons. In spring and fall high concentrations of pollen in the air can set off allergic reactions that cause the lining of the nasal passages in many allergy sufferers to become inflamed and swollen shut. This blocks breathing and makes the person feel miserable. Although nasal sprays may provide instant relief, a rebound effect—swelling of the airway tissues—occurs a few hours later. By this time it may be 2:00

A.M.; the nose is blocked again and the sleeper awakens, uncomfortable as ever and unable to breathe easily. If the hapless allergy sufferer continues using the spray, it has progressively fewer benefits with each use because the body has become accustomed to it.

Another common over-the-counter drug ingredient is caffeine, which is found in pills that encourage wakefulness as well as in some diet pills. In general, diet pills have some stimulant actions, because stimulant drugs somehow suppress appetite.

Fortunately, over-the-counter medications are required by law to list their ingredients on the package. Therefore, a purchaser can ask a druggist or doctor if a nonprescription medicine contains a stimulant that can cause insomnia. Be wary of medications that contain caffeine or other stimulants. The "-amine" suffix on a compound's name can indicate that it might damage sleep quality, although chlorpheniramine, for example, is an antihistamine frequently found in cold remedies that can act as a sleeping pill.

Anyone who has difficulty sleeping after using a nonprescription medication should discontinue its use and, if necessary, see a physician. The doctor might be able to relieve the user's medical problem without upsetting sleep quality. But many people with insomnia have a host of reasons not to sleep, and nasal decongestants are not often considered one of them. Even after a clear-cut incident where use of a cold remedy is followed by a night of bad sleep, many insomnia sufferers ascribe their problem to something else entirely. Thus common over-the-counter drugs are frequently overlooked as causes of insomnia.

HOW PRESCRIPTION DRUGS AFFECT SLEEP

While many prescription medications affect sleep, it is not always possible to tell beforehand whether or not a specific prescription will affect an individual's sleep. Although drugs are meant to relieve physical ailments, they may also have side effects, often on the nervous system, that disrupt sleep. Some prescription drugs are notorious for causing insomnia; others cause it rarely. There is only one reasonably certain test for whether a particular person's insomnia is due to a drug: Did the insomnia start when the person first took it and cease when the person stopped?

Even this test is not 100 percent certain because other causes of insomnia may be present, such as pains or other disturbing symptoms that began when use of the drug started and stopped around the time the drug was withdrawn. Furthermore, the drug might simply be the final straw, when compared with many other causes that may be present, such as caffeine or nicotine, discussed earlier.

Some medications have a relatively high likelihood of disrupting sleep, and their effects are well recognized, as with cortisonelike steroid drugs and most antiasthma drugs. Other drugs likely to lessen sleep quality include so-called beta-blockers, which are used mostly in medications for high blood pressure and sometimes for heart rhythm disturbances, thyroid disease, alcohol withdrawal, tranquilization, and even for suppression of tremors in musicians with stage fright. Many other drugs used for heart rhythm disturbances also interfere with sleep, as do some antidepressant medications taken near bedtime and a few drugs prescribed for migraine headache. Diuretics, commonly used to treat high blood pressure, may disrupt sleep by increasing leg movements, especially among older people.

As mentioned previously, many people take more than one sleep-disrupting drug during the day. For the person who complains of sleeping poorly, this can mean a problematical choice between treating an ailment and getting adequate rest. Of course, sleeplessness itself can worsen many ailments, too. Heart rhythm disturbances, arthritis, and severe depression may get worse with inadequate sleep. So the insomnia patient with significant medical problems who takes potentially sleep-disrupting drugs may face extremely difficult decisions.

Almost any drug can affect sleep. Antibiotics, which have no direct neurological actions, can affect the sleep of some people. Japanese researchers have shown that the commonly used tetracycline antibiotics reduce deep sleep. These antibiotics work by interfering with the synthesis of proteins and thus inhibiting the growth of microorganisms that have protein components. Protein synthesis, however, might be part of deep-sleep functioning, and this might be why tetracyclines affect sleep. These antibiotics may also cause stomach upsets, which could interrupt the quality of sleep.

Antibiotics seldom disrupt sleep in most people, but the point is that you never really know when a drug may interfere with yours. Some unrecognized mechanism may be at work: If a clear correlation persists between poor sleep quality and taking a medication, it may be worth switching to an alternative drug in the interest of good sleep, no matter how rarely the drug disrupts sleep.

There are no simple solutions, but there are ways to optimize the dose and timing of medications—and the routines that affect sleep—to enhance the sleep of patients with chronic disease. This process often requires trial and error to determine the proper drug in the correct dose at the right time under the appropriate circumstances, but it can produce good results. Usually the patient must be willing to make adjustments and to experiment with his or her schedule.

INSOMNIA CAUSED BY ASTHMA MEDICATION

Dr. A. was a medical researcher in her thirties who found herself sleeping more and more lightly. Her condition was due in part to her young daughter, who would cry for attention during the night. Adding to her sleeplessness were nighttime phone calls from colleagues to advise her about problems that developed in her laboratory during the small hours of the morning. After taking the calls, she would get caught up in the situation at hand and then would have even more trouble sleeping.

Her frequent inability to sleep annoyed her deeply, and she decided to work on the problem. To induce slumber, she would read a newspaper or perform some soothing mental exercise, such as imagining a ballerina dancing or a skater gliding over the ice. Sometimes this helped, sometimes it was ineffective.

Television, she decided, might be contributing to her sleep problems. If she watched an interesting program on television, it stimulated her and, she reasoned, made it hard for her to sleep afterward. She stopped watching TV and spent her evenings playing with her daughter and enjoying her husband's company.

Yet the sleep problems persisted. A coffee drinker, she cut out her usual two cups a day. But some things she could not eliminate: her next child, for one. She was four months pregnant, and soon she would be in the latter months of pregnancy, which often cause sleeping problems. The unborn baby kicks, comfortable sleeping positions are harder to find, and the enlarged uterus presses on the bladder, necessitating more frequent nighttime urination. At the same time, Dr. A. was having sinus headaches, and to relieve them she used nose drops, which, as we have seen, can also harm the quality of sleep. When she started to awaken at night with heart palpitations, a rapid, "runaway" heart rate, she went to a sleep clinic.

Ultimately, the problem was not coffee, late-night television, nose drops, or her daughter's late-night crying. Nor was her pregnancy the primary reason for her sleeplessness. The major culprit was a medicine she took for her allergy-induced asthma.

Dr. A. was using two antiasthma medications to prevent wheezing. The medicines acted in different ways. One, called beclomethasone (Beclovent, Vanceril), suppressed inflammation and allergic reactions. The other, albuterol (Proventil, Ventolin), had longer-lasting effects. It widened the breathing passages that were closed by the allergic reactions and also had the side effect of stimulating her nervous system. She and her doctor thought that lowering the dosage might allow her to sleep better, but the question remained how far she could afford to reduce the dosage without risking asthmatic attacks.

Dr. A. had already tried cutting back on the dosage, with no apparent effects. She had not thought much about the *timing* of the doses, however, which is sometimes more important than the dosage itself. So Dr. A. was instructed to reschedule the times she took her medications. Her doctor suggested she take the longer-acting drug early in the morning and use the other anti-inflammatory medication later in the day. That way she would have less trouble sleeping. The new drug regimen cleared up Dr. A.'s insomnia.

As discussed, drugs that act on the nervous system—alcohol, nicotine, or medications—can worsen sleep. People take many drugs precisely because of their effects on the nervous system, but sleep-disturbing side effects accompany their use in people with more fragile sleeping patterns. Prescription drugs, especially those that affect neurotransmission, also affect sleep. Anyone with poor sleep quality is well advised to discontinue drugs that act on the nervous system and, with a physician's guidance, to reduce dosages of necessary prescription drugs to useful minimums. The new pattern of sleep acquired after stopping these drugs long enough to overcome the effects of withdrawal is the starting point for a thorough investigation of disordered sleep.

6

....

Hyperarousal Insomnia

Mark Twain, in his book *A Tramp Abroad,* described how he felt one evening when trying to sleep despite worries that preoccupied him. "I lay there fretting . . . and trying to go to sleep," he wrote. "But the harder I tried, the wider awake I grew." Today we might describe his problem as hyperarousal insomnia. Arousal means susceptibility to stimulation and readiness to act. In hyperarousal, a person is too easily stimulated to sleep well, or even to fall asleep at all. Fortunately, hyperarousal insomnia can often be relieved with proper sleeping habits and relaxation exercises.

Although some people have a distinct tendency to function in a state of hyperarousal, most of us function at a level somewhere in the middle of a range between two extremes: low arousal and high arousal. People who function at either extreme have characteristic traits.

Low-arousal types are unflappable people who do not let things bother them. They are capable of dealing with varied and conflicting stimuli—noises, obligations, decisions, challenges, all bombarding them at once—without becoming flustered or confused. As a rule, low-arousal people do not lose any sleep over the day's problems. Their EEG recordings show why. Low-arousal people tend to display greater-than-average background alpha rhythm in their EEG brain waves. Heightened alpha rhythm indicates that a person is awake but calm. This means his or her composure is difficult to upset.

At the other extreme, high-arousal people would rather handle one task at a time and may become nervous and disorganized if faced with too many stimuli at once. High-arousal people are thinkers and worriers. If something goes wrong at work, they tend to keep fretting and fuming about it long after working hours are over, thus preventing them from falling asleep. They also anticipate problems, thinking in advance about anything bad that might possibly happen in the future. They frequently have some problem on their minds even after bedtime. High-arousal characteristics are reflected in the EEGs of these people. In the background of their EEG records, high-arousal people show much less of the alpha-wave activity that accompanies a calm state of mind. Consequently, they are more easily excited than low-arousal people.

This does not mean a high-arousal personality is necessarily undesirable. In many cases, it goes hand in hand with other, valuable mental traits. People with strongly developed analytical and critical skills, such as researchers, mathematicians, and artists, tend to have high-arousal personalities.

High-arousal people make good workers in a wide variety of jobs because they are conscientious, sensitive to subtleties, and capable of detailed, accurate work. They take their work seriously, do it thoroughly, and leave little room for error or failure. These people are often thoughtful, introspective types. Although they may get rattled easily, they are sensitive to others.

But because they concentrate intensely on their work, they can become upset when many simultaneous demands are made on their time and attention. Our very stimulating world can easily become unnerving to them. Many high-arousal people suffer from insomnia, becoming so keyed up by the end of the day that they are unable to unwind and fall asleep.

For some hyperaroused individuals, the less they sleep, the harder it becomes to fall asleep. They complain that they are too tired to fall asleep. It sounds improbable, but there is some evidence that such a complaint is valid. In fact, sleep deprivation can make some people excitable and nervous rather than fatigued. This agitation combined with hyperarousal interferes even more with sleep. Eventually the upset and hyperaroused patient may sleep for a while, but the constant tendency toward insomnia continues.

Hyperarousal insomnia has been difficult to understand and diagnose because it has no specific diagnostic criteria. The personality profile described earlier seems to be an underlying tendency like a personality trait. But beyond administering standard psychology tests, personality has not yet been investigated much in insomnia, certainly not enough to allow firm connections to be made. Besides, there may be many hyperaroused people who sleep well and never consult with doctors at sleep clinics.

The analogous type of insomnia in the American Sleep Disorders Association (ASDA) official classification is called persistent psychophysiological insomnia. The ASDA hypothesized that psychophysiological insomnia was due to internalized psychological tension and rapid conditioning (or "learned" insomnia) in which insomnia became a conditioned response to bedtime. Dr. Peter Hauri tested these hypotheses at the Dartmouth Sleep Disorders Clinic at Dartmouth College, however, and found many fewer psychological abnormalities than expected, with no confirmation that these insomnia patients had been conditioned to associate insomnia with their bedtime behavior or surroundings. Furthermore, they did not have any more tension, as measured by muscle electrical activity, than comparable people who did not suffer from insomnia. Patients did tend to repress and deny things more than others, so the ASDA's original concept of this type of insomnia patient might be on target: Some of these patients are unduly tense.

Dr. Anthony Kales at the Hershey Medical Center has vast experience with sleep problems and believes that internalized psychological tension characterizes much of the insomnia in patients he sees. It may also be that insomnia and tension both derive from some third factor such as hyperarousal, rather than one causing the other. Moreover, sleep deprivation itself can cause tension in some people, and vice versa. Some patients with insomnia of no obvious cause also seem normal on the psychometric tests that measure distress. In the end, all the explanations for other types of enigmatic insomnia—for example, the tension-conditioned insomnia and psychological distress hypothesized previously—do not apply to many insomnia patients.

For insomnia sufferers who lack obvious causes such as biological clock disorders, psychological disturbances, and drug use, the mechanisms that cause insomnia remain unknown. This situation will probably continue for some time. The amount of research into insomnia is disproportionately small compared with that of other sleep disorders such as narcolepsy and sleep apnea, in which more definition of the problem is possible, and positive findings are easier to uncover. In *The Diagnostic and Statistical Manual of Mental Disorders,* the official diagnostic classification of insomnia having no cause or explanation is referred to as "primary insomnia." Someday medical science may find that primary insomnia has another cause, but right now all practitioners can do is present their best guesses. Hyperarousal probably accounts for much primary insomnia.

The sleep clinic of Brigham and Women's Hospital collected stories hyperarousal patients told about themselves, using them to create the questionnaire on page 102. The clinic also measured the alertness of the patient's nervous system with the aid of electrophysiological tests, quantitative analysis of the EEG, and cortical auditory evoked potentials derived from the evoked potential test. In it, an electrode is pasted to a person's scalp and the voltage of an electrical potential ("brain wave") is measured after a beep tone is played into his or her ear. This measures how immediately responsive the nervous system is. For most people, the louder the tone, the larger the brain wave. In hyperarousal patients, the greater-than-average height of some of the waves correlated with their high scores on the questionnaire. This meant that the behaviors that hyperarousal patients noted in themselves might well be connected to the greater responsiveness of their nervous system.

Also, the questionnaire scores correlated with how much

alpha-rhythm activity there was in the EEG. This was measured performing a mathematical operation on the EEG called *Fourier transformation*. This technique separates the different types of brain waves—alpha, delta, theta, and others (see chap. 1)—on the EEG. The Fourier transformation is distinctly different from the usual eyeball inspection of the EEG because the brain waves that are the most visible (alpha during wakefulness and delta during deep sleep) are not mixed in with the other rhythms. For example, with the traditional method of inspection, delta activity is concealed; after Fourier transformation researchers could see how much delta activity there was even during wakefulness.

According to the Fourier transformation, the hyperaroused person also shows more alpha rhythm. This is not much of a surprise, really, since alpha rhythm goes with wakefulness, and the hyperaroused person is more awake. But with the traditional method of reading the EEG, the hyperaroused person actually seems to have less alpha than the person who is awake but calm. Noisier EEG activity that corresponds to the very awake state of having one's eyes open obscures the underlying alpha rhythm on the EEG paper printout.

More practically, the hyperarousal patients all scored in a different range on the questionnaire when compared with people who had no insomnia, even though only three of the questions pertained directly to sleep. The responses to other questions seemed to indicate personality traits that went along with hyperarousal. The different range of scores also suggested that the hyperarousal trait was not one end of a normal spectrum; instead, something about these insomnia patients was qualitatively different from those who slept normally, and this difference spilled over into other areas that did not involve sleep. Researchers at the sleep clinic feel that this questionnaire might help diagnose hyperarousal insomnia.

Here is the questionnaire. To find out whether you might be in the hyperarousal category, rank the statements from "not at all" to "extremely," as they apply to you. An explanation of how to score the questionnaire appears at the end of the chapter.

Hyperarousal Questionnaire

Check each statement as it best relates to you:

	Not at all	A little	Quite a bit	Extremely
My mind is always going.	____	____	____	____
Bright lights, crowds, noises, or traffic bother me.	____	____	____	____
I cannot take naps even if I try.	____	____	____	____
I tend to anticipate problems.	____	____	____	____
I take things personally.	____	____	____	____
I get rattled when a lot happens at once.	____	____	____	____
I have trouble falling asleep.	____	____	____	____
I am a cautious person.	____	____	____	____
In bed at night my thoughts keep going.	____	____	____	____
A sudden loud noise would cause me a prolonged reaction.	____	____	____	____
I am overly conscientious.	____	____	____	____
Caffeine affects me strongly.	____	____	____	____
When things go wrong I tend to get depressed.	____	____	____	____

Some thoughts re- turn too often.	___	___	___	___
I take a long time to make deci- sions.	___	___	___	___
I get tearful easily.	___	___	___	___
I keep thinking about some things long after they happen.	___	___	___	___

Hyperarousal insomnia can be relieved in most cases, usually by removing sleep-disrupting influences from a person's life and lowering his or her arousal level near bedtime. Arriving at an individualized program can take some trial and error, as the following examples illustrate.

INDIVIDUALIZED TREATMENT OF HYPERAROUSAL INSOMNIA

Mr. A. was a 36-year-old teacher who had suffered from insomnia for many years. His insomnia rarely abated. Most often, he had difficulty falling asleep at night. He thought something was wrong with him, and that increased his anxiety and made sleep even more difficult.

His sleeplessness was especially bad when something had disturbed him emotionally during the day. An argument at school would keep him upset and preoccupied long into the night. When he did fall asleep, even the slightest sound would awaken him and keep him awake for a while.

Anything related to Mr. A.'s profession obsessed him. Gifted in math, he had a talent for computer programming and had recently taken a course in assembly language, which he worked on compulsively. If the solution to a programming challenge eluded him at first, he could not stop thinking about it until he had the answer, even if it took all night.

The school where he taught granted him a sabbatical to work

full time on developing software for learning–disabled children. Mr. A. saw the project as a rare opportunity for these children's self-expression, and it became one of his major reasons for living.

A brief vacation from the project helped. Mr. A. slept better when the tempo of his life slowed down a bit. Even nighttime noise disturbed him less. (He was lucky in this respect, because vacations have just the opposite effect on many hyperaroused people: the new and unfamiliar stimuli make it harder to sleep.) When the vacation ended, the ordinary stresses of daily life had Mr. A. lying awake in bed again night after night. And now that he lacked a rigid schedule of morning classes, he began sleeping late, thus further reducing his chances of falling asleep at a regular bedtime.

Mr. A. tried treating himself, and to some extent it worked. He avoided caffeine. Jogging seemed to tire him out, but he found that, near bedtime, it had the opposite effect. He achieved good results from special relaxation techniques. Sometimes he augmented these techniques by soaking in a hot bath or applying a hot towel to his forehead. Occasionally he indulged in a massage. He also tried drugs, including marijuana and tranquilizers, but he disliked using chemicals and decided to seek help at a sleep clinic.

Mr. A. hoped to avoid psychotherapy; the thought of probing deeply into his own motivations made him uncomfortable. He preferred to "treat symptoms rather than causes," he said. Yet he also displayed a keen understanding of his own attitudes. Fortunately for Mr. A, the high-arousal personality that caused him trouble also brought relief. People who can focus their attention well, as high-arousal people can, also tend to respond to hypnotism. Thus, Mr. A. responded well to relaxation tapes, which he liked much more than most patients do. This was Mr. A.'s own version of what psychologists call *guided imagery,* using mental pictures invoked by sound to steer oneself toward a desired state of mind. He continued the relaxation exercises as well. Gradually he relaxed enough at bedtime to fall asleep.

In the last analysis, Mr. A.'s sleep problems were a matter of control—more accurately, the *sense* of control. He felt confident when he was in command of a situation and nervous when he wasn't. This need for control was the key to solving his sleep problems. His treatment depended on exercising and on being disciplined about his relaxation exercises and his sleep/wake schedule. Mr. A. had command over this regimen, as opposed to relying on the effects of drugs, which made him feel ill at ease.

The first time he took a nap in the afternoon was a milestone. Before long, his sleep disorder became progressively less of a concern. Soon Mr. A. realized how radically he had changed. He said it felt "weird to know how to get to sleep every night."

A quite different case required similar but still individualized treatment. Ms. B. was a slim, athletic woman who worked for the international division of a large corporation. For 15 of her 38 years, she had required two hours or longer to fall asleep at night. Even then she sometimes awoke in the early hours of the morning without getting enough sleep.

Her sleep problems had their origins in the previous day's activities. If something unusual or upsetting happened during the day, it occupied her thoughts far into the night. As a result, she dreaded going to bed. On weekends and holidays she allowed herself to sleep late in the mornings.

Ms. B. tried the time-honored remedy of exercise, as Mr. A. had. She ran 4 to 5 miles a day and skied frequently in the winter. But exercise was not the remedy for her. If she ran for 40 minutes or more, she enjoyed the euphoric "runner's high," but if she ran in the evening, it took her even longer than usual to fall asleep. Skiing worked no better. When she had an especially invigorating day on the slopes, the exhilaration made her even less likely to fall asleep that evening.

Ms. B. tried everything she could think of to relieve her insomnia. She gave up caffeine. She tried psychotherapy, hypnosis, and relaxation training. Each were effective for about two weeks, then she found herself lying sleepless in bed again at night.

For a mysterious insomnia problem like Ms. B.'s, internists may prescribe antidepressant drugs empirically. Antidepressants do help some people sleep, sometimes immediately. Many of these drugs act on multiple neurotransmitters that affect sleep, and this may explain their sedative effect in some people. In Ms. B.'s case, however, the antidepressant pills had unanticipated strong effects. One pill knocked her out until noon the following day. The same thing happened when she tried another type of antidepressant.

When Ms. B. went to a sleep clinic, her problem was diagnosed as hyperarousal insomnia. She described herself as a careful, scrupulous, effective worker, and as someone who was always thinking, the characteristic traits of the high-arousal personality. For treatment, she kept a sleep chart, discontinued her daily glass of wine with dinner, and maintained a strict schedule of going to bed at midnight and arising at 7:00 A.M. She was instructed to run no later than 7:00 P.M., and to run at a regular time each day rather than on an irregular schedule.

She also did progressive muscle relaxation exercises (see p. 109). These exercises take time to learn, and several weeks may pass before substantial relaxation is achieved. It took time, but Ms. B. overcame her hyperarousal insomnia. She would no longer lie awake at night, trying to escape her nagging thoughts, and even when she woke up in the middle of the night, getting back to sleep was not difficult.

Like many other patients who have lived a long time with hyperarousal insomnia, Ms. B. was astounded at the change in her life. She was rising early in the morning, but awakening more refreshed. How, she asked, was this possible on her new, seemingly abbreviated sleep schedule? Actually, her sleep was not abbreviated at all. Her prescribed sleep schedule had been based on her average total sleep time per day, but the new schedule eliminated the late-morning sleep that had upset the regularity of her daily sleep rhythm.

It seemed too good to be true, and for a while Ms. B. feared that in the end this treatment might be no more successful than earlier attempts to cure her insomnia. But the regimen worked. To her immense relief, Ms. B. had finally found the dependable sleep she needed. Her basic personality had not changed. She remained a high-arousal person, but progressive relaxation training had taught her how to deal with the sleep problems that often go with such a personality. During the day she could take advantage of the positive side of her high-arousal personality to carry out her work, and evenings she could turn off the flow of high-arousal thoughts and achieve a refreshing night's sleep. Ms. B. became an advocate of relaxation training.

TREATMENT FOR HYPERAROUSAL INSOMNIA

More and more often, patients at sleep clinics include high-arousal people who have treated themselves successfully for hyperarousal insomnia using simple, commonsense techniques and have come to the clinic for reassurance that they are doing the right thing. High-arousal people tend to be bright and perceptive, and they realize they can do much for themselves to overcome hyperarousal insomnia.

Many try vigorous exercise to induce sleepiness, and get mixed results, as Mr. A. and Ms. B. did. Exercise affects sleep differently in different people. Exercise stimulates, refreshes, and increases metabolic rate and neurotransmitter levels. All these effects are likely to further stimulate a high-arousal person. On the other hand, exercise also raises body temperature and uses energy, thus leading to deeper sleep hours later, when temperature drops again and people who have exercised feel more fatigued. In short, in high-arousal people, exercise interferes with sleep at first, then promotes sleep later. Those who find that evening exercise damages sleep would do better to work out in the morning or afternoon.

If exercise does not work, there are other techniques the hyperarousal insomniac may try. One approach is to turn down the body's metabolic thermostat, or to reduce the signals that set the rate at which the body uses up food energy. Generally speaking, regulating the metabolic thermostat from higher to lower means that sleep comes more easily.

Metabolic rate is impossible to control by conscious effort. A person cannot simply reset the metabolic thermostat a notch or two down, because humans are warm-blooded animals whose survival normally depends on keeping a constant body temperature, and a steady metabolic rate is a must. But the body can be tricked into making a metabolic downshift. Just before bedtime, the person with hyperarousal insomnia can fill a tub with very warm water (about 105°, or more if bearable) and soak in it with most of the body submerged. (*Caution:* This may not be good for people with some heart problems; they should check with their physicians before trying this technique.) Deep, old-fashioned tubs work best. Soon body heat starts to build up because, surrounded by hot water, the body cannot cool itself either from sweating or from circulating more blood to the skin, which is usually cooler than the body's core and from which heat can usually radiate.

Internal temperature soon rises. Feedback mechanisms in the hypothalamic area of the brain act to restore body temperature by dilating blood vessels in the skin, producing sweat and turning off adrenaline-caused responses ordinarily present during states of excitation. As discussed in chapter 3, the hypothalamus regulates another basic vital function, body timing. The hypothalamus also affects body temperature, and in a hot bath where sweating and other short-term adjustments cannot restore normal temperature, metabolic rate may be turned down. This may reduce the level of arousal as well. In any case, experimenters have observed that people who raised their body temperature by soaking before bedtime had more than usual deep sleep during the night.

People with hyperarousal insomnia should soak for about 20 minutes, but take care when standing up because some may feel faint and giddy. Body temperature should rise a degree or two. After this temperature rise, sleep should come more easily as the body temperature falls slowly over the next hour.

Tub soaks are not a guaranteed cure for hyperarousal insomnia by any means. Fainting can occur because blood has been redirected to vessels near the skin, thus lowering blood pressure and causing insufficient blood to reach the brain when the person stands up.

One patient claimed the giddy, unstable feeling she experienced at the end of the soak helped her sleep because it made all the day's anxieties drain out of her. Some patients who have tried tub soaks report that they felt uncomfortably hot after getting in bed beneath the covers. One patient had to lie unclothed on top of the bed for a while to cool off. One might think this cooling would undo the effects of the soak, but evidently it did not.

THE PROGRESSIVE RELAXATION EXERCISE

The progressive relaxation exercise briefly mentioned earlier was devised by Dr. Edmond Jacobson and is sometimes called Jacobson progressive muscle relaxation. It is best to start practicing the technique during the daytime, when sleep is not an immediate concern. It is essential to perform the exercises at a regular time and in a quiet, solitary place where you can lie down and do the relaxation procedure properly. Don't lie down where a ringing telephone, spouse, child, or pet can interrupt you. The technique should be done in five stages, as follows.

1. Become aware of gravity. Lie on your back on a wide bed or a soft rug. Close your eyes. Uncross your legs. Your hands should lie limp at your sides, so that no part of your body has to bear the weight of any other part. Trust gravity alone to keep you in place.
2. Concentrate on your feet. Picture your feet relaxing completely. Think of nothing but your feet. Envision them as blocks of stone, needing no direction from you. Some people imagine their feet as masses of warm, wet towels—lying there. Other people imagine warm, wet towels draped comfortably over their feet, or that warm sunshine or other heat is focused on their feet and relaxing them. Eventually your feet should feel as if they are on their own. Let them take a rest.
3. Relax upward, body part by body part. As soon as your feet are thoroughly rested, move the relaxation through your legs using the same techniques. Focus on the left calf, then the right calf; the left thigh, then the right

thigh. Repeat the relaxation with your hands, your right and left forearms, your left and right upper arms. Let each part become loose, limp, and relaxed. Feel tension draining out of each part of your body. Think of your breathing. It feels good to fill your chest with air. Breathing in is a pleasure and to exhale takes no effort; you can "relax" the air out of your chest. Some people think of releasing tension with each exhalation. Continue this procedure through the trunk and shoulders until your whole body below the neck is thoroughly relaxed.

4. Relax your head. Send the feeling of relaxation upward from your body through all the many muscles of your head—the muscles on the back of your neck, jaw muscles, eyelids, eyebrows, and forehead. Let your jaw hang open a bit. Ignore noises or other distractions. Devote all your attention to relaxing your head.

5. Take inventory. When you have finished relaxing your head, see if there are any remaining parts of the body you have forgotten to relax or that you want to relax more. If so, you might try this trick to relax them: Tense them as much as you can, then let them go. For example, make a tight fist, then let it relax. For many people, the result is better relaxation, though it may not work for everyone. Some people find that tensing any muscle aggravates arousal, just the thing you are trying to avoid. If tensing recalcitrant muscles makes you more awake, then stay with the progressive relaxation technique exclusively and do not use muscle tension to relax.

To score the Hyperarousal Questionnaire on page 102, count every answer in the "Not at all" column as zero. In the next columns, count 1 for "A little," 2 for "Quite a bit," and 3 for "Extremely." A score above 26 indicates hyperarousal.

7

....

Depression and Phobias and Their Effects on Sleep

About 20 percent of women and 10 percent of men suffer a bout of severe depression during their lives. In addition to its other effects, depression commonly causes loss of sleep. Some cases of depression resolve themselves when the problems that caused them vanish. But other cases of depression are more deeply rooted in the body and mind. Left undiagnosed and untreated, depression may cause sleep loss for much of a lifetime. Fortunately, depression and its attendant sleeplessness and sleep-related problems can be relieved.

Like depression, phobias, which are irrational fears, may also cause sleeplessness; they too can be relieved with proper diagnosis and treatment.

Virtually everyone, at one time or another, loses sleep over life's ordeals. Sadness about one's own or a close friend's misfortune, such as a sudden loss of a job or a serious health problem, may temporarily interfere with one's sleep. In most cases, sleep soon returns to normal when the individual starts to cope with the situation.

Many people, however, have serious problems with depression. A chronically depressed person can't rebound easily from life's disappointments and losses. A depressed person's mood

111

goes down and stays down for extended periods. Severely depressed people are unable to take interest or pleasure in life. Nothing friends or loved ones can do is any consolation. Depression sufferers may feel incapable, worthless, and that they are always in the wrong and/or would be better off dead. Sleep seems to offer the depressed person a brief respite from his or her agonies, but sleep remains elusive. For some, tormenting thoughts crowd their minds as soon as the bedroom light goes out, making sleep almost impossible. For others, sleep comes rapidly at bedtime but lasts only a few hours. After that, the depressed person remains miserably awake. Some depressed people suffer from the opposite problem, they sleep too much, which is a condition known as hypersomnia. Clinical depression and its related sleep disturbances may last for months and even years. Connections between depression, the body's clocks, and neurotransmitters may explain why insomnia often and hypersomnia sometimes accompanies depression.

REACTIVE VERSUS ENDOGENOUS DEPRESSION

To understand how depression affects sleep, it's necessary to first understand the types of clinical depression. Two principal kinds of depression are now distinguished from each other: *reactive* and *endogenous*. Both kinds of depression disturb sleep. Reactive depression is what its name implies: depression that occurs in reaction to distressing events. The death of a family member, divorce, or the breakup of any other close and valued relationship often causes reactive depression. A spell of reactive depression may last several months, depending on the sense of loss.

Despite the discomfort and pain reactive depression causes, it often indicates sound mental and emotional health. Something might be wrong in a person's emotional makeup if an event such as a loved one's death did not cause reactive depression. Reactive depression—another name for it is grief—is characterized by overwhelming sadness, lack of enthusiasm, and the inability to enjoy things or concentrate on one's work. Mourning the loss becomes the key to overcoming reactive depression—gradually coming to terms with one's loss and then turning to the world again and getting on with life.

Endogenous depression ("arising from within") occurs for no obvious reason and has its roots in the person's psyche. It seeps up insidiously and invades a person's thoughts and emotions until it has a complete hold.

Certain personality types seem unusually prone to endogenous depression. These sufferers are likely to be self-sufficient, principled persons who hold themselves to high standards and try their best at everything they attempt. These people have many traits in common with the high-arousal personality described in the previous chapter. What exactly causes endogenous depression remains uncertain. There seems to be a genetic component involved, because studies have revealed that chronic, severe depression can run in families.

Until recently the physiological factors behind depression have been little investigated. Certain diseases actually cause depression in a high proportion of those afflicted—diseases involving high levels of steroid hormones, or brain pathologies due to stroke, tumors, or injuries in locations that affect emotion (especially the frontal lobes on the right-hand side of the brain). Some drugs might even cause depression as an unwanted side effect. Evidence gathered years ago would indicate that depression could have physical causes, but doctors have generally assumed that most depression was brought on by deficiencies or devastating losses during childhood—insufficient love and acceptance, or the death of a parent—with inevitable damage to psychological development.

This theory does not account for why some people who suffer severe losses in childhood manage to overcome them and function very well, while others become severely depressed. There are probably physical differences in the physiological mechanisms of mood that underlie these outcomes. Possibly these differences are genetically determined.

During the 1950s, medicines were discovered that could relieve depression. The idea that medication could relieve serious depression was novel, but it implied there was some biochemical reason for at least some depressions. This surprising finding set off decades of research to find out how the treatment worked. Now, years later, more is known about the physiological causes of depression.

The first physiological theory about endogenous depression involved neurotransmitters that antidepressants affect, called *catecholamines.* As noted earlier, certain neurotransmitters play a role in regulating normal mood. Catecholamines can cause depression if their levels in the brain fall too low, and can cause mania if their levels rise too high. Another neurotransmitter, serotonin, which plays an important role in the regulation of sleep, seems to account especially for the emotional pain of depression, as distinguished from energy loss, disinterest, and inability to concentrate. The brains of suicide victims have been found to contain abnormally low levels of serotonin compared with people who died in accidents. Perhaps the actual levels of neurotransmitters are only part of what determines mood. The sensitivity of nerve cells to them may also play a role. The concept of nerve-cell sensitivity arises because antidepressants increase the action of relevant neurotransmitters soon after they are taken, but it usually takes weeks for the depression itself to lift, a course that parallels changes in nerve-cell sensitivity to the neurotransmitters.

But there is evidence to contradict the neurotransmitter theories; for example, some antidepressant drugs do not alter neurotransmitter levels. Therefore, other physiological mechanisms may exist for depression. There are many other substances, such as hormones and neuropeptides (a peptide is a short chain of amino acids), that seem to influence mood. The most famous neuropeptides are the *endorphins,* the body's natural equivalent of morphine, which are secreted especially in the event of physical pain.

Hormones such as cortisol can affect mood. Cortisol normally aids the actions of other hormones and is secreted in greater amounts whenever the body suffers some kind of distress. One major action of steroids (cortisol-like drugs) is to suppress inflammation, which is the body's general reaction to injury. (Sometimes the inflammatory reaction is greater than needed or inappropriate for the circumstances, and therefore steroid drugs are used widely in medicine to control inflammation.) Some people who take steroids become very depressed and suffer from sleeplessness. Some people become elated and sleep less than normal but tend not to complain about it due to their elevated mood.

Estrogen and *progesterone* are two other hormones that affect mood. Estrogen decreases the action of two enzymes, *catechol-o-methyltransferase* and *monoamine oxidase*. These enzymes inactivate catecholamines after they are released from the nerve endings during neurotransmission. So estrogen tends to increase the actions of catecholamines. Lower estrogen levels, such as those found during menopause, may increase depression. Estrogen and progesterone may also affect the blood level of tryptophan, the amino acid precursor of the mood-altering neurotransmitter serotonin. It is hard to determine exactly how these hormones affect mood. They may influence the neurotransmitters, which affect not only mood but also sleep, appetite, the perception of pain, and energy—clinical ingredients in depressive syndromes. Progesterone has significant sedative effects in some individuals, and both hormones affect the sex drive.

With all this complexity of possible mechanisms, and the individuality of nerve-cell-type profiles, the effect of hormone pills given for birth control or for symptoms of menopause becomes unpredictable. Birth control pills can create depression and the sleeplessness that accompanies it in some users. Estrogen replacement clears up depressive symptoms in some menopausal women. Such evidence suggests that lack of estrogen actions or lower progesterone levels may be involved in worsening depressions, especially those that occur after menopause or in the final days of a woman's menstrual cycle. Thyroid hormone imbalance, as discussed previously, can also induce depression and sleeplessness.

Another physiological factor that affects mood is the action of the internal biological clocks. These internal clocks have a profound effect on sleep, as discussed in chapter 3. Of the body's two internal clocks we described, the one that controls the 24-

hour cycle of highs and lows in body temperature also controls the peaks and valleys in cortisol levels. In endogenously depressed people, the schedule of this internal clock seems to become disconnected from that of the other clock, which times the sleep/wake cycle. Researchers find that the peak of cortisol levels in the blood, which occurs normally around 8:00 A.M., takes place much earlier in endogenously depressed people, perhaps around 3:00 A.M., when many depressed people awaken. Thus the usual timing for cortisol's highest levels (and probably for many other physiological functions as well) is thrown off. The earlier that the cortisol peaks, the more depressed the person feels.

The minimum level of body temperature for the day, which normally occurs around 4:00 A.M., also comes earlier in endogenously depressed people. This means not only that the usual pattern of physiological highs and lows throughout the day is changed, but also that the synchronization between the body's two internal clocks is disrupted. The cause of this disruption is not known, but one reason may be insufficiently strong signals to the body about what time of day it is, as caused by irregularities in mealtimes or exposure to daylight, for example.

Researchers at the National Institutes of Health (NIH) have found that getting depressed people to arise early in the morning can actually make their depressions disappear, at least for a while. This procedure realigns the peaks of the sleep/wake cycle with those of the body temperature–cortisol cycle or, more basically, resynchronizes the two internal clocks.

Very early rising, to the point of partial sleep deprivation, has a marked antidepressant effect on some people. They find they can avoid serious depression by arising very early once or twice a week. Conversely, people commonly become depressed after sleeping late in the mornings. Even if they feel fine awakening at 7:00 A.M., some will feel poorly if they fall back asleep and awaken at 9:00 A.M. NIH researchers have reported that some depressed people who took antidepressant drugs, but found no relief, finally felt better when they were also made to get up earlier. Therefore, synchronizing the body's clocks by matching the sleep/wake cycle to the body temperature–cortisol cycle may have a practical therapeutic effect on mood.

A physiological connection between internal clocks and mood may explain why yet another physiological factor bears on depression: bright light. It was well-known in the nineteenth century that the countries of northern Europe had higher rates of suicide than the Mediterranean countries. The difference was attributed to a stern ethos sometimes associated with the Protestant religion. But twentieth-century statistics indicate that in South America, where practically everyone is Catholic, suicide rates also increase with distance from the equator. Apparently the more brightly lighted climes have fewer suicides. Some depressed people, especially those who feel worse in the winter, can find relief by exposing themselves to bright light in such a way that the light lengthens their days. Thus, they sit before very bright lights during the dark of the early morning and the late afternoon and early evening, extending their "daylight" hours.

The physiological causes for depression just mentioned—neurotransmitters, hormones, and the internal clocks—may be interrelated. Steroid hormones may augment the actions of some neurotransmitters, while some neurotransmitters that seem to affect mood also regulate the body's clocks and strongly influence sleep. Thus there may be a whole physiological mood-regulating system that was previously unknown and from which much about depression can be inferred.

DEPRESSIVE SYMPTOMS

Although the ultimate origins of endogenous depression are still murky, at least the progress of the condition is well understood. Slowly, over an extended period, sufferers find their moods darkening. They may become impatient and demanding or lose interest in usual pleasures. Little problems that once seemed insignificant soon appear unsurmountable. Sleep is disrupted, often in a characteristic way. The endogenous depressive is likely to start awakening too early in the morning. One study of severely depressed patients revealed that 87 percent of them had problems with early awakening. Sometimes this early awakening can give way to fitful sleep the whole night long. These sleep disturbances are primary diagnostic indicators of depression. Before long the sufferer's distress becomes obvious, with symptoms such as agitated speech, frequent complaints, temperamental outbursts, increased sensitivity to lights and noise, and, in some cases, crying spells. Physical symptoms may appear, including headaches (or other pains), constipation, diarrhea, and weight loss due to diminished appetite. The sufferer may interpret this weight loss as a sign of some other disease, such as cancer. It is common for a chronically depressed person to fear that he or she has a terminal or life-threatening disease but to conceal this fear from his or her physician.

Denial is also a characteristic of endogenous depression. The depressive person refuses to admit that anything is seriously wrong. "I've just been working too hard," he or she often says, "I need a vacation." Unfortunately, vacations cannot cure endogenous depression. Depression may end in tragedy, a life of misery, or suicide.

Of course, such a tragic fate is not inevitable. Endogenous depression and the troubled sleep that accompanies it can be remedied. Sometimes treatment requires both patient and physician to overcome formidable obstacles, notably the fear of the very drugs that promise a cure. Many depressed people get well on practically any antidepressant treatment. Even relief of serious, long-term depression is possible in a large majority of cases. But the patient must be identified as depressed before the treatment can begin. Epidemiological surveys estimate that a little over 2 percent of the population is suffering major, endogenous depression. Many are undiagnosed, misdiagnosed, or untreated. The biggest task in treating depression is to find practical screening methods to identify depressed people who can be helped by medical treatment.

SCREENING FOR DEPRESSION

Although it is still difficult in some cases to decide whether a depression is endogenous or reactive, recent progress is encouraging. There remains no sound physiological method to determine if a person suffers either form of depression. Tests that outline neurotransmitter metabolism, special techniques that measure brain waves, and methods using X-raylike radioisotopes to analyze the metabolism of parts of the brain during various mental tasks show promise as diagnostic tools. The main development has been a rebirth of interest in treating depressed-mood symptoms themselves, such as sleeplessness, rather than possible psychological triggers. Other advances have centered on methods to validate standardized questionnaires and use them for research.

The need for consensus about depression among interested parties, from government statisticians to insurance companies, has spurred interest in standardized criteria for diagnosis and has led to the formulation of official diagnostic classifications for it.

The standardized criteria for depressions of various sorts have been published by the American Psychiatric Association (APA). Using standardized criteria, physicians can more easily study an individual's symptoms to diagnose his or her depression. Of course, offical lists of depressive symptoms may not be the best or the only way to diagnose endogenous depression. For instance, the doctor's own appraisal of the patient or a history provided by the patient's spouse may be crucial. Nonetheless, the checklist of symptoms can serve as a screening device to detect patients with depression who otherwise might be missed and thus go unhelped.

In the near future, more sophisticated lab tests will be available to outline the disorders of patients suffering some kinds of insomnia and depression. Measurements also may help determine what type of depression a person suffers from and the best treatment for it. In our times, however, diagnosing depression is more art than science. Most often we must make a guess about which antidepressant treatment is right for a particular patient based on the symptoms suffered. As mentioned previously, depressed patients sleep poorly because of physiological changes that disturb their internal clocks, moods, and sleep quality. Thus, chronic sleep problems serve as a red flag for depression. The following case illustrates how treatment for insomnia can play a major role in the treatment of depression.

INSOMNIA TREATED WITH ANTIDEPRESSANTS

Ms. A. was a 40-year-old social worker who had suffered insomnia on and off since childhood. In recent years her problem had grown worse, and now she found herself unable to remain asleep for long periods of time. She felt constantly depressed and cried throughout sessions with her therapist.

Sleeping pills helped her get to sleep for a night or two after she began taking them, but then they ceased to be effective. Yet when she stopped taking the pills, she suffered even worse insomnia than before. In addition, she felt guilty about resorting to medication, and her self-reproach made sleep that much more elusive. Psychotherapy had made her better able to fall asleep at bedtime, but she also began to awaken more often in the middle of the night. Ms. A. even resorted to hypnosis at one point, but it didn't work. (Hypnosis usually does not help people with insomnia because the focused intensity of the trance state is contrary to the unfocused relaxation that precedes sleep.)

Ms. A. avoided many habits that disrupt sleep. She neither smoked nor drank coffee, and she ate reasonably and exercised regularly. Even so, many factors were working against her. She had the classic high-arousal personality and some serious family problems—an unhappy marriage that had ended in divorce and an alcoholic son.

Finally Ms. A. went to a sleep clinic for help. She made regular visits to the clinic to discuss her sleeping problems, but it was over a year before she accepted a prescription for doxepin (Adapin, Sineqnan), an antidepressant drug. Within two weeks, her sleep problem disappeared. "My whole system responded!" she said. Now she was getting eight hours of good sleep each night. Doctors did not prescribe antidepressants earlier in her treatment because she was not ready to accept them.

As mentioned earlier, Ms. A. was loath to take pills to relieve her condition, and when she did take sleeping pills, their ineffectiveness convinced her even more that any medication was no answer to her insomnia. Also, she believed that her insomnia, even if it was rooted in her personal problems, was beyond her control. In her words, the insomnia had "a stubborn life of its own."

Ms. A. went to a sleep clinic requesting psychotherapy, but she already had arranged a large array of treatments she thought would relieve her insomnia. She had seen a psychotherapist to deal with her psychological problems, a behavior therapist to teach her relaxation techniques, and a hypnotist to attempt relief by hypnosis. Now she wanted a sleep doctor to add psychotherapy slanted toward possible causes of her insomnia.

Also, she took part in various workshops that covered relaxation methods and psychological techniques such as "reframing," in which the patient supposedly learns to view insomnia in a new and more productive light. Reframing teaches the patient to see insomnia not as a series of sleepless spells in the middle of the night but rather as a fresh opportunity to do things while awake. Reframing might help others who need to change their attitude toward a problem, but in this case, it shows how well-intentioned but nonspecific treatments do not relieve endogenous depression.

There are plenty of practitioners available with appealing theories and claims about every kind of psychological symptom, and who offer diet, prayer, psychotherapy, or reframing, but nonspecific treatments confuse the person with an undiagnosed endogenous depression and may lead him or her to an expensive array of "treatments," as Ms. A. had discovered. Of course, sometimes these methods do bring relief, and endogenous depression in some cases does disappear spontaneously. Much of what helped Ms. A. was building enough trust and rapport with her doctor at the clinic so she could accept the idea that endless self-analysis and self-reproach were not the answers. Eventually, her resistance to using antidepressants diminished, and she agreed to start taking them. Partial relief was almost immediate.

About three weeks after beginning the antidepressants, however, Ms. A. suffered a setback. She had been cutting back on her sleeping pills while beginning to use antidepressants, and in time had stopped taking the sleeping pills altogether. Ordinarily, a gradual discontinuation of these pills causes little in the way of withdrawal symptoms, but Ms. A. was exceptionally sensitive to drug withdrawal and found herself unable to sleep.

Her physician advised her to resume taking the sleeping pills but at a reduced dosage. The goal here was to get her off the sleeping pills entirely and onto the antidepressant, but to do so in a way that would reduce her fears and self-doubts and prevent drug-withdrawal insomnia. Overcoming those obstacles was much more important than following strict pharmacological rules, which might have meant stopping one pill before starting the next.

This strategy allowed her to get off sleeping pills entirely. Soon Ms. A. was also free of insomnia. She felt better than she had in a long time, and agreed to remain on the antidepressant for a year. Had she accepted the antidepressants in the first place, she would have been spared months of needless suffering. But she had to be prepared psychologically to accept the treatment, or she simply would have given up. She became an example of how, in the treatment of sleep disorders, a slow approach can actually be the most effective.

LENGTH OF TREATMENT WITH ANTIDEPRESSANTS

Antidepressants are not like sedatives or painkillers that at some dosage exert predictable action on anyone who takes them. Some people, perhaps most, feel only side effects from antidepressant drugs.

Most people who benefit from antidepressants can take them for a year and then gradually get off them without relapsing. A year is a long time, but those who discontinue antidepressants after only three or four months have a high rate of relapse—about 15 percent. Therefore, a longer treatment period seems worthwhile and appears to sustain relief in a way that is necessary to prevent relapse. Possibly the nervous system develops more sensitivity to its neurotransmitters during this time, but the actual mechanism is unknown.

UNTREATED DEPRESSION

The media often reports about the tragedy of untreated mental illness. Untreated depression is just as noteworthy because it can be remedied, and therefore many people are suffering needlessly from it. Unfortunately, depression is often overlooked in the diagnostic process.

A 32-year-old clinical psychologist suffered from crying spells, paralyzing ruminations, indecisiveness, and insomnia. She had completed four years of psychoanalysis and was now in psychotherapy once a week. She had consulted a psychopharmacology expert and had begun taking an antidepressant, despite strong opposition from her family, who disapproved of psychoactive drugs.

At first, it appeared her family was right. She proved highly sensitive to the antidepressant and promptly became oversedated. A single antidepressant pill made her so groggy that she had difficulty responding to her own patients. After taking two such pills, she could hardly get out of bed.

After this unpleasant experience, she vowed never again to take antidepressants. But insomnia continued to vex her. She tried the basic measures—giving up caffeine, keeping a sleep chart, and so forth—but her insomnia persisted. For 17 months, she had been treated with the aid of instruction, support, and psychotherapy, plus a combination of two sedatives, neither of which helped her appreciably. At last, on her doctor's urging, she agreed to try antidepressants again.

Someone who felt groggy from a single antidepressant pill was surely going to require special treatment. In her case, it consisted of dosage by the drop: she started taking an antidepressant in liquid form, a few drops at a time. At 16 drops, she achieved reliable sleep for the first time in 10 years.

RESISTANCE TO ANTIDEPRESSANTS

Why do so many people resist taking antidepressants? The reasons include fear of side effects, the wish to avoid dependence on drugs, and the reluctance to appear ill. Yet these motives do not completely explain widespread negative attitudes about antidepressants. Many people who shun antidepressants are happy to take sedatives.

Possibly a cultural factor is at work here too. In our secular society, the mind has largely replaced the ancient concept of the soul as the symbol of the essence of being. Since antidepressants and other psychoactive drugs affect mood, some people are afraid that pills will alter their very being—cost them their souls. They would rather struggle unaided against a mental disorder than risk becoming another person under the influence of a drug. This attitude is costly in every sense of the word. It can cost the depression sufferer sleep, productivity, and peace of mind. And it is sad to contemplate the many cases of depression-related insomnia that go untreated because the sufferers believe that using any drug is a sin. In fact, antidepressant drugs only change symptoms, not one's basic personality.

PHOBIAS AND SLEEP PROBLEMS

For years, phobias have been thought of as the intense anxiety that one attaches to particular objects or places, the sight of which might cause a panic attack. It gradually became clear, however, that being generally anxious and having phobias and panic attacks were not one and the same. For example, many phobias are triggered by objects and situations that cause fear in most people, such as the sight of a snake or looking down from a great height. Humans may have evolved instinctive fears of some things because they might prove fatal on first encounter.

Some people suffer panic attacks with little provocation. During routine activities such as shopping or sleeping, they may be seized with a feeling of life-threatening terror accompanied by all the physical reactions that go with it: shaking, trembling, profuse sweating, racing heart, shortness of breath, pains, or other symptoms. Panic attacks often interrupt sleep. A panic attack is particularly upsetting when it occurs in public, where one may feel alone and helpless; some people become afraid to leave their homes. This disorder is called agoraphobia, an unreasonable fear of public places. Public speaking, a common phobia, is one of the most difficult tasks for some panic patients. They might find themselves in such a situation without warning, for instance when they could unexpectedly be asked a question in a room full of people.

The intensity and suddenness of panic attacks suggests some physiological abnormality may be involved. Researchers have been able to induce panic attacks in patients by various physical means, such as infusions of lactic acid (a substance produced by working muscles) or by having the person inhale carbon dioxide (another metabolic byproduct). New scanning devices indicate that in panic patients, some areas in the emotional control system of the brain have higher-than-usual metabolic rates. Measuring metabolic processes such as glucose utilization or the blood flow in various areas produces a picture of important dynamic processes in an individual's brain. Before long, these new measurements may help us better understand panic disorders.

Certain medications appear to relieve panic, and not simply because they have a calming effect. One tranquilizer, alprazolam (Xanax), seems especially effective against panic if compared with other tranquilizers. Alprazolam is a member of the family of tranquilizers most commonly used today, the benzodiazepines. Its relatives include diazepam (Valium), triazolam (Halcion), flurazepam (Dalmane), lorazepam (Ativan), and many others. Many of the differences among these drugs involve the speed with which they are absorbed into the nervous system— and how fast they are excreted. The ones more rapidly excreted are less likely to cause a drug hangover but more likely to cause withdrawal problems. Alprazolam seems qualitatively different from its relatives, however: it may relieve depression and often relieves people with panic attacks. Although the other medications relieve anxiety, they do not prevent panic attacks. These large differences suggest that alprazolam has more actions on the nervous system than its relatives. Some antidepressants that are not sedatives also help prevent panic attacks.

Most phobia treatments require some kind of contrived behavioral routine, such as subjecting the patient gradually to the stimulus that provokes the phobic symptoms, or the support of a group of similarly phobic people who might attempt to endure the panic-inducing condition together. The patient may do relaxation exercises, and then imagine aversive conditions such as boarding an airplane or getting into a dentist's chair. Starting a relaxation treatment is a matter of trial and error as well as the patient's preference. Some people prefer the longer progressive relaxation exercises, others like the simplicity of easily learned meditation routines.

INSOMNIA CAUSED BY PHOBIA

Mr. A., a businessman in his fifties, would awaken in the middle of the night gasping for breath, trembling, and feeling panic and palpitations. He counted his heart rate at 120, almost double the normal resting rate during sleep for a man his age. His problem seemed due partly to being overweight and to the eight to ten beers he drank daily. Yet even after he stopped drinking and lost more than 40 pounds, he continued to complain of fitful, restless sleep, and he felt insufficiently rested during the day. He also felt anxious when anticipating certain situations, such as speaking in public or traveling in the middle lane of a superhighway. Once, when asked to address a convention of a large national organization, he refused. He explained that important people would be there, and he would feel like an imposter addressing them.

Even though Mr. A. had stopped drinking, he said he would fall apart if he ever got too far away from what he called his "support system": a cooler full of beer that he carried with him everywhere. Before an airplane flight, however, he would consume a six-pack or more. On these trips, he felt safer when accompanied by a company employee, a family member, or a friend.

His fear of public speaking and travel had hurt his generally successful consulting business. He turned down a large government contract because he felt he would fail if forced to endure the kind of public scrutiny the contract would involve. He also feared the long-distance air travel, which would have been unavoidable.

On examination at a sleep clinic, Mr. A. was friendly, talkative, and cheerful. He was willing to discuss uncomfortable subjects related to his condition. Tests revealed no obvious psychological basis for his problem, and there were no signs of depression. Sleep-laboratory recordings showed he had no sleep apnea, which can also cause someone to awaken frightened from sleep. But Mr. A. did suffer from agoraphobia as a result of his fear of having a panic attack in public.

Mr. A. was prescribed an antipanic drug, alprazolam, which overcame the panic rapidly. Only a small dose was required, as it sometimes is when the effects of a medication are specific. It was amazing: suddenly Mr. A. could drive the turnpike without worries and sleep without fear of panic attacks. He was even able to speak in public, although he was never thrilled at the prospect. Nevertheless, he could live free of ghastly anticipation.

The case histories in this chapter demonstrate that many instances of sleep disorders related to psychological problems can be treated. Perhaps the most tragic aspect of such cases is that so many of them are avoidable yet remain untreated. That is why the diagnostic process should consider psychological factors if no physiological disorder exists to disturb a patient's sleep. Investigating the possibility of depression or some other mental suffering may save the insomnia patient years of misery and fruitless treatment.

Many patients with insomnia assume that anxiety causes their problem and hope that their treatment will consist mainly of psychotherapy. But there are substantial disadvantages to overlooking other possible treatments.

For example, the sleep-hygiene methods mentioned in case histories earlier—arising at regular times, giving up substances that affect the nervous system, exercising regularly, practicing progressive relaxation, and so forth—are so inexpensive and effective compared with psychotherapy that they should be attempted first (see chap. 11). Also, psychotherapy alone does not seem to relieve insomnia. Note that two of the patients described earlier had been disappointed that psychotherapy failed to relieve their symptoms. Psychotherapy is often long-term examination of complex psychological problems that spring from the assumptions, values, and hopes that make a person what he or she is. Insomnia, though complex, is nonetheless just a symptom and can be relieved in a short time—certainly more quickly than psychotherapy can undo complicated problems such as an inability to get along with people or a chronic sense of failure.

However, some people whose sleep problems have been properly evaluated find they cannot follow prescriptive instructions for remedying the problems. For example, almost everyone will have trouble giving up smoking. Others will find it tremendously hard to stop sleeping late in the morning. Patients trying to cope with such problems may need practical psychotherapy to help them develop good habits (see chap. 14).

8

....

Insomnia and
Other Sleep Disturbances
in Older People

Insomnia is a common problem among older people and has many causes, from reduced daytime activities and growing symptoms of illness to the widespread use of hypnotic drugs that are intended to encourage sleep but instead may affect its quality. Although sleep is more solid in youth than in later years, insufficient sleep is not inevitable. Most older people sleep well. And in most cases, when sleep fails, the individual can take effective action to ensure an adequate amount of good-quality sleep.

Misunderstanding the sleep difficulties of older people has handicapped research in this field. One common misconception is to think of older people as a homogeneous group when it comes to sleep-related problems. On the contrary, older people are a diverse group in almost every respect, and in many cases, studies of sleep disturbance in older people have had to be further refined to make the subjects under study easier to categorize. For instance, one study may deal only with hospital patients or with retired professionals, groups whose characteristics are clearly defined, enabling researchers to make certain assumptions about the people studied. It is tempting to apply the results of such limited surveys across-the-board to anyone over 65. It is also a mistake to do so, because there is no typical sample of sleep disorders in the older population.

There is also the widespread and incorrect assumption that poor sleep is an inevitable companion to aging. Many people might have an older relative who complains of not being able to sleep at night. Physicians treating sleep disorders in older people often hear the same refrain: "I have trouble sleeping at night, but that's just because I'm old." Advanced age by itself, however, does not mean that one is naturally condemned to troubled sleep. This misconception prevents many treatable cases of insomnia from being diagnosed and relieved.

HOW SLEEP CHANGES WITH AGE

The amount of daily sleep lessens gradually throughout childhood, from the 16 hours or more of the newborn to the 8 to 8½ hours of the teenager. For the adult, total sleep per day becomes increasingly an individual matter. Although the average amount of sleep remains about 7½ hours throughout adulthood, older people obtain more of this amount from daytime naps and less from nighttime sleep. There is great variation around the 7½-hour average. Some people obtain 4 hours or even less per night, while others might require 9 hours or more daily. We tend to adhere to an average number of sleep hours, although some of us might sleep 7 hours and 15 minutes one night, 7 hours the next, 7½ hours the next, and so forth. Still, total sleep hours per month tend to be the same from month to month.

Many older people who complain about insomnia are told simply that old people need less sleep. This fails to address their complaint that something is wrong, regardless of any averages, and it contradicts the fact that researchers observing older people and collecting sleep charts found that older adults often obtain just as much sleep as younger ones.

Although sleep quality does not deteriorate suddenly when a person turns 65, it is true that the quality of one's sleep tends to wane with age. An older person's sleep patterns represent a culmination of trends that developed over his or her lifetime. As a person ages, he or she gradually experiences less very deep sleep, a slight reduction in total sleep time, and more nocturnal waking periods that disrupt sleep.

These changes are well under way long before a person reaches 65. A 30-year-old person, on the average, gets less than half as much very deep sleep (stage 4) as a 20-year-old does, and awakens twice as often during the night. But such changes are much more apparent in an older person, because the trends they represent have had so long to develop. Whereas a 20-year-old may spend only 5 percent of the night awake in bed, a 70-year-old is likely to spend about 15 percent of the night in a wakeful state. (This figure increases to about 20 percent at age 85. In other words, it is normal for an older man or woman to lie awake for about a fifth of the night, or roughly an hour and a half.) The greater wakefulness of later years accompanies the drop in very deep sleep, so that someone in the eighth or ninth decade of life may be completely deprived of the deepest slumber.

It also follows that in later years people need progressively longer to fall asleep. The person who falls asleep within 8 or 10 minutes at age 30 may require more than 15 minutes at age 70. The older person also needs more time to return to sleep once awakened in the middle of the night. Thus if some problem such as arthritic pains from changing positions disturbs an older person's sleep several times a night, he or she will suffer several wakeful periods of perhaps 15 to 20 minutes, which can add up to a significant loss of quality sleep.

Although a significant reduction in REM sleep at advanced ages might be expected, older people appear to get as much REM on the average as their children and grandchildren do. A 1972 general study of REM sleep indicated that people between ages 16 and 79, taken as a group, display the same amount of REM sleep, about 22 percent of total sleep time.

Many elements of the sleep EEG show changes that parallel the subject's increasing age, but the earliest and most outstanding change in sleep is decreased amplitude in slow-wave, or delta-wave, activity. This type of EEG rhythm signifies the deepest sleep of the night, as discussed in chapter 1. The EEG of a typical child, teenager, or adult shows the prominent highs and lows of slow-wave activity in the record. By about age 65, however, the so-called delta waves have become shorter and, in some cases, may be only one-half as high as they were half a century earlier. The decline in delta-wave amplitude is greater around age 65 and afterward. This change is more pronounced in men than in women, who tend to show very little difference in delta-wave activity between the teen years and their 60s. Whereas changes in delta-wave amplitude are part of a progressive, overall decline in the amount of brain-wave activity with advancing age, changes in other EEG frequencies are less marked.

There are "cycles" or repeated patterns of sleep during the night, as shown in the somnograms in chapter 1. These cycles are composed of alternations between deep or medium sleep at the beginning and REM sleep at the end of each cycle. Three or four such cycles make up a night of sleep. The cycles are longer toward the beginning of the night and longer during youth, when a larger portion is actually deep sleep. As deep-sleep periods grow briefer, the cycles grow briefer and become interrupted more frequently by wakeful periods, resulting in the lighter, more broken sleep of advancing age.

One study of institutionalized women at a Boston rehabilitation center revealed an unexpected feature of sleep in older patients. The amount of nighttime sleep correlated with the amount of daytime sleep. That is, the more the patient remained awake at night, the more she also remained awake during the day. This was a surprise that contradicted the widely held assumption that increased sleep time during the day means less sleep at night. The positive correlation between daytime and nighttime sleep suggests that the older patients had a general tendency toward sleepiness or wakefulness that was present throughout a 24-hour period.

INSOMNIA INCREASES WITH AGE

The subject of insomnia in people over age 65 has undergone extensive statistical research. One 1962 survey of over 2,400 adults in Scotland revealed that sleep disturbances increase dramatically with age. The study showed that complaints of seriously disrupted sleep increased steadily with each succeeding decade of life, until by age 75 about one-third of the people surveyed were frequently afflicted with fitful sleep. One-third may seem an excessive figure, but it has been confirmed by other studies in Great Britain and the United States. One English study found that more than half the healthy people over age 70 suffered from sleep irregularity.

An American Cancer Society survey of sleep problems among older people revealed that nonspecific sleep disturbances—for which no particular cause could be established—increased in linear fashion over the years, from 8 percent for men and 14 percent for women in their thirties, to 17 percent of men and 31 percent of women in their early eighties. A separate study of older men and women in Florida produced comparable figures.

Advancing age alone does not suffice to explain the decline in sleep quality that many older citizens experience. As noted earlier, most people over 65 have acceptable sleep quality, and a few individuals in their seventies and beyond sleep as well as they ever did. Yet insomnia is more common at this age, and sleep specialists have proposed a wide variety of explanations.

NERVOUS SYSTEM DEGENERATION

The cerebral cortex, the outermost layer of the brain, loses nerve cells steadily over the years. The result is a decline in both brain size and interconnection among brain cells. As the total number of cells decreases, so does the number of links, or synapses, among the cells. A typical person loses over 100,000 brain cells a day, until upon reaching the seventies, he or she has lost about 20 percent of the cells in the cerebral cortex. This loss is not a steady process. Rate of degeneration appears to reach a peak in a person's fifties, and not all portions of the brain lose cells at the same rate. Some areas are affected at a faster rate than others.

Such structural deterioration of the brain has been linked in older people to changes in alpha rhythm, or background rhythm, of the EEG. The waking EEG background rhythm becomes slower as people age, from about 10 to 12 cycles per second in the young to 8 to 10 cycles per second in the old. This change may reflect nerve-cell loss in the cortex, although the death of nerve cells may not be the only factor at work. Other age-related changes such as decreased blood flow to the brain, which reflects diminished brain metabolic rates, may explain slowing in EEG activity. At least two studies suggest a link between cerebral blood flow and EEG alpha rhythm. Generally speaking, a higher-frequency background EEG rhythm means more alertness during the day. Higher alpha-rhythm frequency also accompanies preserved REM sleep at night.

These conclusions are supported by the findings of a 1977 study in which 22 people, ages 82 to 97, had their EEG monitored as they went about a normal day's activities. The subjects were fitted with telemetric equipment that allowed them to move around freely, thus eliminating the need to remain in the laboratory. (Laboratory-bound subjects would have been restricted in their activities, and this would have affected the outcome of the experiment.) The study showed that age and the waking frequencies of the EEG were indeed correlated with amount of wakefulness, sleepiness, and naps.

More research is needed to determine the precise connections between age-related EEG changes and sleep quality, but two things seem clear. First, degenerative changes in the central nervous system appear to be responsible for much of the decrease in sleep quality observed in older people. Second, aging by itself does not account for the degeneration, because many older people sleep soundly and show little deterioration of the nervous system. In fact, sleep quality depends not so much on a person's age as on his or her health. Studies of older people show that intactness of the nervous system, determined by learning tests or blood-flow studies, predict sleep quality better than a person's age. The same is true for breathing disorders during sleep, the incidence of which generally increases with age. This occurs because of structural degeneration of the lungs and also because with age there's less fine-tuning of the breathing control mechanisms. Healthy older people actually have few such problems, demonstrating again that for sleep quality, health means more than age.

Even when older people sleep well, however, they may remain more susceptible to sleep-disrupting influences than younger people. They are more easily awakened by noise and are more sensitive to caffeine's sleep-robbing effects.

BLADDER PROBLEMS

Many older people find their sleep disturbed because they must urinate frequently during the night. In men, this often occurs because of irritation caused by an enlarged prostate, but any irritation of the bladder or urinary tract can have the same effect on sleep for both men and women. Frequent urination itself can lower the threshold for the urinary reflex, an automatic reflex that creates the urge to urinate when urine reaches a certain volume in the bladder.

Frequent urination during the night can cause loss of sleep in older people because it takes longer for them to fall asleep once awakened. To decrease nighttime urges to go to the bathroom, a person can reeducate his or her urinary reflexes by slowly and progressively delaying urination whenever the urge arises during the daytime. Most people can delay urination for a few minutes. A person who must go to the bathroom immediately or lose bladder control has more than a urinary reflex problem, and should have the problem investigated by a physician.

A person can progressively lengthen intervals between urinations as follows. For one week, every time he or she feels the urge, urination should be delayed 15 minutes. The delay interval should be increased to 30 minutes the second week, and thereafter gradually increased until the person can wait up to 90 minutes by about the sixth week. After the 90-minute interval has been reached, the person should drink extra water in the morning, gradually increasing the amount from one to four glasses—about a quart—over a month's time. At that point, the urge to urinate during the night should be less frequent because "bladder training" has reeducated the urinary reflex; the bladder is now able to hold more urine than before. Restricting fluid intake in the evenings may further prevent sleep disturbances, but bladder training might make such dehydration unnecessary.

SLEEP-CLOCK DISORDERS

The internal clock that maintains a rhythm for the human sleep/wake cycle all through life takes its cue from external timing information such as the light/dark cycle and regularly timed social events. In later years the sleep clocks seem more vulnerable to disruption, resulting in damage to sleep. In short, older people are more prone to a sleep/wake cycle that can be at odds with our society's normal night-day schedule.

The body's internal two clocks—the one that runs the sleep/wake rhythm and the other that governs the temperature rhythm—rapidly become desynchronized when people are put in isolation, cut off from all evidence of the time (see chap. 3). They sleep and awaken at whatever time of the day they wish. In a 1975 study that isolated experimental volunteers for 8 to 10 days, 21 percent of time-isolated subjects ages 17 to 33 showed desynchronization of their circadian rhythms, compared with 100 percent of older subjects ages 44 to 69. Removing our external pacemakers shifts complete control of the body's timing to our internal clocks, and the timing of sleep and wakefulness in older people departs much more easily from normal coordination with other body rhythms.

The more frequent sleep-clock troubles in older people may be due to a lessened sensitivity to external pacemakers such as the light-dark cycle or the social schedule that keep our sleep timed normally. It is also possible that the link between the two internal clocks grows weaker during old age, so that they constrain each other's timing less. The weakened link may be one example of an overall decline in the efficiency of the body's regulatory mechanisms with advancing age.

The sleep clock of an older person may also be upset by lack of social contact. Socializing with other people is one of the principal influences on our circadian rhythms; humans tend to be awake and active when those around them are awake and active, and to rest and sleep when other people in the immediate environment are doing the same. An older person, however, may have this influence removed, at least on occasion. He or she may have fewer opportunities for social contact as family members move away, old friends die, or retirement removes the person from the working world. Some older people are detached from others and become withdrawn, especially when illness occurs. Thus they become more self-centered and lose much of the daily stimulation of wakeful days and sleep-filled nights that maintains the rhythms of life. When deprived of normal social contact or social interest, a person's sleep clock may then be prone to upsets, because one of its strongest regularizing factors—interaction with other people—is missing.

The modern world has provided passable substitutes for human companionship in the form of radio and television. Scheduled programs such as soap operas, news programs, and talk shows may serve as a daily reference point for a solitary older person and thus help prevent the sleep clock from straying too far from synchronization. Television provides a surrogate "society." Its regular schedule can give the isolated viewer both a bearable alternative to the fast pace of modern society and a timer of sorts for his or her sleep clock.

REGRESSION

Generally speaking, regression means a psychological return to an earlier way of life. This is an almost universal phenomenon among older people and is often invoked to explain changes in sleep patterns, especially the increasing frequency of daytime naps. Older people are prone to taking short naps during the day, thus regressing to the pattern of daytime sleep/wake rhythm commonly observed in early childhood.

Figure 10 is a schematic diagram of sleep as it progresses throughout the life span. Like everything else, sleep changes most during the childhood years. By 10 years of age, daytime naps are rare, and in adulthood sleep is shorter. When sleep quality worsens, however, people can regress backward along this developmental path. First they may go to bed earlier, as they did in late childhood, and then they might take a regular nap, a routine of earlier childhood.

Of course, there are whole societies that take afternoon siestas, reflecting the physiological remnants of development present in all of us. But when the individual takes multiple naps, both in the morning and in the afternoon (as shown for the one-year-old), some major illness is usually present. No matter how ill a person becomes, the first-stage pattern is not found in adulthood, nor even much beyond one year of age.

Regression in the psychological sense is a more or less defensive tactic, a response to overwhelming challenges. In regression, a person goes back to the routines of an earlier time when life was supposedly simpler. Sometimes regression means a psychological tendency to seek magical relief from discomfort with little personal effort. A good example is the wish for a perfect sleep drug.

DRUGS

The widespread, some would say pandemic, use of hypnotic drugs by older people can lead to damaged sleep patterns. Some drugs, for example flurazepam (Dalmane), have been found to result in the buildup of metabolites that linger in the bloodstream for long periods and may help to bring on drowsiness during the day. Another drug, triazolam (Halcion), is so short-acting that unlike most other sleeping pills, it has been totally excreted from the body by bedtime the day after it was taken. This rapid elimination of the drug from the body causes slight symptoms of drug withdrawal in some people. As in other

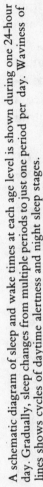

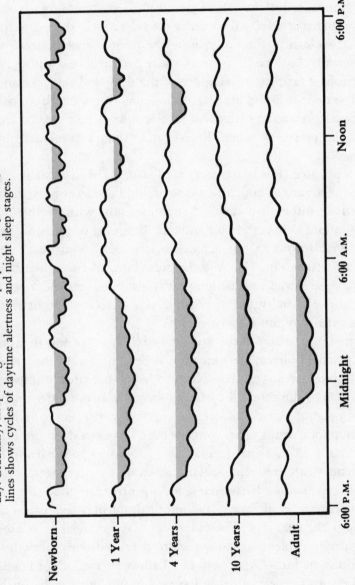

A schematic diagram of sleep and wake times at each age level is shown during one 24-hour day. Gradually, sleep changes from multiple periods to just one period per day. Waviness of lines shows cycles of daytime alertness and night sleep stages.

Figure 10 Schematic representation of sleep patterns over a human life span.

sedative withdrawal periods, a person may feel more anxious.

Research orthodoxy at present prefers short-acting sleeping pills to long-acting ones. Some research points out, however, that the excretion time alone determines less about a drug's next-day hangover effects than other considerations: the proportion of fat to lean in the body, how the drug is metabolized, and above all, the dose. In general, older people have a higher proportion of fat that stores more of the drug and then continues to release it into the bloodstream. Some drugs that have complicated metabolic paths will take longer to be excreted from an older person's system. Illness can prolong and increase drug effects.

In practice, research averages of patients who actually have insomnia vary so much that doctors find different pills are optimal for different patients. Sometimes pills with troublesome reputations help certain individuals. But most of the time, people with insomnia can achieve better sleep with good sleep hygiene (see chap. 11). And the point remains that when sleeping pills are used to treat long-term insomnia, the older person can suffer a multitude of possible side effects, some of which he or she may not be aware.

Ironically, many of the drugs taken by older people to induce sleep actually harm sleep quality, depending on the individual. Longtime use of sedatives tends to lessen the already impaired function of the cerebral cortex observed in many older people, thus making already troubled sleep still worse. Sleep induced by hypnotic drugs often contains even less deep sleep and more waking periods than normal sleep does. So for many older patients with frequent, persistent insomnia, hypnotic drugs probably do more harm than good. Deprived of good sleep and hung over, chronic users of hypnotic drugs may feel listless and groggy the next day. The older user may not even be aware of this drug problem and may seek to correct it with more drugs or think of him- or herself as a listless person. Coordination and responsiveness, already lessened in old age, can be further impaired by sleeping pills. Daytime falls and injuries may result.

One disturbing effect of hypnotic–drug use among older people is a tendency toward occasional episodes of unusual agitation and confusion, when the drugs suppress inhibitory functions of the cerebral cortex. Unfortunately, physicians treating agitated episodes in older patients do not always recognize the cause and instead compound the problem by prescribing still more hypnotic drugs or sedatives during the day. This may occur because the older patient (or his or her family) insists on more medication. It might also take place in a hospital or nursing home where an agitated resident disturbs other residents. In one 1972 study, about one-sixth of older patients who were admitted to mental hospitals were cured of their behavioral disturbances when sedatives and antidepressants were discontinued.

It is plain to see that treating older people with hypnotic medications can harm their sleep and behavior. Less obvious, but just as significant, is that sleeping pills simply humor an older person's regressive tendencies. He or she might use pills as a tool to recapture the passive, dependent state of early childhood—use them, in other words, as a substitute for mother love. In times of distress, many people might tend to regress to a less mature, less responsible stage of life. Most older people have suffered some loss—of strength, energy, loved ones, or status. The tendency to regress is so great that the drug user will continue taking the medication even if told of the harm that the pills may cause.

This is not to say that the use of sedatives is totally harmful. Hypnotic drugs certainly offer benefits to some users. It may be argued that even drugged sleep is better than complete sleeplessness. A physician cannot be dogmatic about the pros and cons of sedatives in this context, because every person with insomnia must be considered as an individual, and it must be determined whether use of such drugs is justified. In general, use of sleeping pills may be more justified for the person who remains generally healthy, self-sufficient, and employed or who regularly helps others. The healthier person is more likely to have the reserves to tolerate inevitable disadvantages from use of sleeping pills.

DISEASE

The pain that many older persons experience from illness such as angina or arthritis can interfere with sleep. The hospitalized older patient may be especially susceptible to sleep disturbance due to illness or its symptoms, hospital noise and dislocation, and unpleasant methods of treatment. Sometimes medications, particularly those used for asthma or hypertension, can disrupt or preclude sleep.

Of course, many factors bearing on sleep disturbance in the older person, such as chronic illness, are not within the individual's control. But a patient can still do everything possible to lessen the effects. He or she can follow diligently whatever treatment is needed, get rid of aggravating factors such as smoking or obesity, and generally aim to live as healthfully as possible despite the pain of illness. Unfortunately, regression does much to impair a person's active resolve to cope with difficulties.

THE EFFECTS OF LINGERING IN BED

Sometimes older people regress psychologically by remaining in bed too long each day. Studies based on questionnaires or direct observations of older people reveal that many of them remain in bed long beyond their total sleep times. They may lie there 10 hours or more, fruitlessly hoping for 8 hours' sleep. But they probably drift in and out of light, fitful sleep and make their bed into a place for frustrated wakefulness rather than refreshing sleep.

A 1987 report from the Montefiore Sleep Disorders Center in New York indicates that lying in bed too long makes a person with insomnia feel worse. In the report, insomnia patients who spent too much time awake in bed were persuaded to reduce drastically the total time they actually lay in bed each day. They started with a maximum of four and a half hours in bed per day. Fourteen of the forty-nine patients who began the study dropped out because they could not bear this initial period. Those who remained reported the total time they lay in bed and the time they actually slept each day. When they were able to sleep at least 90 percent of the time they were in bed (this was very easy for people spending only four and a half hours in bed), their time allowed in bed was increased gradually until they spent an average of six and a half hours in bed nightly. That may not sound like a great amount of sleep, but after completing the program, patients reported substantial improvement. They felt less drowsiness and fatigue during the day, despite their brief times in bed.

WHAT YOU CAN DO

These findings suggest that many people who spend much of their time lying awake at night are setting themselves up for more fatigue, rather than less, the following day. So the older person seeking better sleep might wish to try remaining in bed only for the time he or she sleeps. If you sleep only five hours a night, for example, you might stay in bed only from midnight to 5:00 A.M. If you cannot stay awake until midnight and must go to bed at 9:00 P.M.(thus having to rise at 2:00 A.M.), you have a sleep-clock problem as much as an insomnia problem. You can sleep, but at the wrong time. Try restricting your in-bed hours to the total number of hours you need per day. As sleep quality increases, you may be able to stay up later. Otherwise, in order to stay up later, you might try adding a nap after lunch, including the naptime in your count of daily total sleep.

Many people resent the idea that they should reduce their in-bed time to help their insomnia. But results like those from the Montefiore clinic show that this approach may be worth trying.

There is much else you can do for sleep disturbance, starting well before old age, to minimize troubled sleep as you get older. Your main goal should be to avoid withdrawing from society or losing interest in life in general. This only brings on the isolation and consequent sleep-cycle disruption mentioned earlier. We cannot offer a rigid, specific prescription for reordering your life to optimize sleep quality, but here are some steps that older people may wish to consider taking for better sleep. Remember that sleep is after all a part of life; the happier and more satisfying your life is, the better you are likely to sleep.

1. Take care of some business every day outside the home. Changing your environment, even by so little as a walk around the block to the store, increases contact with the world and its infinite stimulation. Some readers might find this suggestion obvious and trivial—or even insulting—but some older people do actually refuse to leave the house.

2. Exercise regularly. The exercise need not be strenuous (a daily walk is a good start in most cases). Even moderate exercise, if done regularly, improves muscle tone and cardiovascular fitness. Before beginning an exercise program, consult with your physician. If pain, shortness of breath, or some other physical problem makes exercising difficult, have the problem treated and after consulting with your physician begin regular exercise, supervised by a specialist in fitness.

3. Become involved in something that interests you. A hobby can boost the spirit. Community, church, and volunteer activities can serve the same purpose.

4. Tend to your own interests. Live for your own interests, and your other family members will probably be much happier to see you do so. Refrain or desist from living vicariously through your children and grandchildren.

5. Don't be quick to relocate. Many older people think they can achieve a happier life in some other part of the country, and move there, thinking they will find solace in a new environment. In many cases, however, all they do is swap one set of problems for another. You may do better to stay where you are and cultivate relationships with friends, family, and neighbors you already know.

6. Evaluate yourself for problems mentioned elsewhere in this book. If you have a sleep-disturbing problem with medications, alcohol, or tobacco, depression, or some

other problem, do something about it. Think about the problem as something that can be overcome. Talk with your doctor about it, and have your doctor help you or help you find help. Your doctor has a referral network or may know more about national organizations and advocacy and self-help groups that can address your needs. It might be uncomfortable initially for you to attend an Alcoholics Anonymous session or other self-help groups, but you are sure to learn a great deal. The American Lung Association often has lists of groups that can help you stop smoking. A good psychiatrist can provide an assessment for depression or even for a problem that produces feelings of hopelessness. Taking a first step itself will make you feel as if you can actually do something more than regret.

Above all else, remember that aging does not necessarily mean you are sentenced to insomnia or any other sleep disorder. Learn to accommodate the aging process while removing sleep-robbing influences from your life.

9
....

Childhood-Onset Insomnia

One of the most perplexing sleep disorders is childhood-onset insomnia. Children sleep so soundly, as a rule, that any disturbance of sleep usually has little effect. Teenagers are able to keep irregular schedules, drink lots of coffee, lead frenetic lives—and still sleep well. But sometimes insomnia begins in childhood: the younger a person is when insomnia begins, the worse it tends to be. The child seldom complains of insomnia, and feels fine during the day, even though his or her parents may think it odd to find their child reading comic books by flashlight under the blankets at midnight. This sleeplessness may remain tolerable through the high school years and even into college. But by the third decade of life, childhood-onset insomnia usually brings on daytime sleepiness and misery.

Why a few children sleep much less than others has not been studied extensively. Observations by Dr. Peter Hauri, now at the Mayo Clinic Sleep Disorders Center, suggest that slight neurological problems, manifested by a history of reading or behavior problems in childhood, subtle reflex changes, or slight but nondiagnostic EEG findings might lie behind childhood-onset insomnia. These signs can indicate minor disturbances in the function of the neocortex. Although such disturbances would be barely perceptible during the day, they would worsen sleep quality at night.

Some specialists in sleep disorders have considered childhood-onset insomnia as a special type. Yet the insomnia that begins in childhood, like adult-onset insomnia, is likely to be a number of different kinds of sleep disorders lumped together under one name. Patients with childhood-onset insomnia exhibit a wide range of symptoms and are helped by a correspondingly wide variety of treatments. One patient with severe childhood-onset insomnia displayed an unusually high percent of stage 4 sleep and was treated successfully with opiates, while another patient with a diagnosis of childhood-onset insomnia showed an extremely low percentage of stage 4 sleep and required treatment with trazodone (Desyrel), an antidepressant medication.

It would clarify things if stage 4 sleep was definitely connected with the actions of either opiates or trazodone. In fact, nerve cells that react to opiates or to serotonin, the neurotransmitter whose action is stimulated by trazodone, probably do influence how much stage 4 sleep a person obtains. But the sleep-regulating system has so many parts and interconnections, any of which presumably can go wrong, and the current tools for studying the system are so crude by comparison, that specialists can observe only these extreme examples when they occur and hope to transcribe them into a theory that would guide further research.

So it is misleading to think of childhood-onset insomnia as a single disorder with consistent causes, symptoms, or treatments. The patients mentioned above demonstrate how greatly two individual cases of childhood-onset insomnia can differ.

CHILDHOOD-ONSET INSOMNIA
TREATED WITH OPIATES

Mr. A., a mechanic in his midthirties, had never been able to get much sleep at night. At age 5, he slept only about 5 hours per night, and by age 18 his total daily sleep time had fallen to only 2½ hours. This inability to sleep began to cause him serious psychological problems at age 16. He became the bad boy of his high school and was constantly involved in car wrecks and difficulties with the law. By age 22, his near-sleepless nights left him in a terrible state of agitation. He would pace around the room in a frenzied manner. After days of little sleep, he would suffer visual hallucinations as well. His family found him difficult to deal with and ostracized him.

Like many other persons plagued with severe insomnia, Mr. A. sought relief in alcohol. The results were unfortunate. He would drink himself into unconsciousness, from which he eventually would awaken foggy-headed and unable to function. Then he began to use heroin and discovered that it brought him relatively refreshing sleep. For the next 10 years, Mr. A. maintained his heroin habit, juggling the dosage to accommodate his sleep requirements and his tolerance for the drug, and taking frequent drug holidays to prevent habituation to the drug. Mr. A. might have continued this regimen for years more, but economic problems intervened. He had a car-parts business that was wiped out in a recession. With his business gone, Mr. A. no longer had enough money to purchase his heroin, and his insomnia returned.

Beset once more by sleeplessness, Mr. A. turned to an outpatient clinic for help. There he tried many drugs to relieve his problem, including minor tranquilizers and more than a dozen other substances that might sedate him or work somehow on his sleep. In constant misery, he slept hardly at all and was unable to do much of anything except eat and walk. At night he would walk for miles, and the town police on night beats came to know this troubled figure roaming in the darkness.

Mr. A. remained so agitated that he was unable even to keep a sleep log for himself. Finally he was hospitalized and was hardly a model patient. Unkempt and foul-smelling, he stalked around his room chain-smoking cigarettes and complaining of minor inconveniences. Nonetheless, his doctor was able to examine him closely and discovered, by having a nurse look in on him every half hour, that he slept only 11 hours out of a 116-hour monitoring period. The nurse's sleep chart showed long horizontal lines indicating continuous wakefulness, broken only here and there by narrow "ravines" that stood for brief snatches of sleep. A polygraph record of a night's sleep showed that Mr. A. was awake for hours after the recording, which was started shortly after midnight. Mostly he was talking with the laboratory technician and smoking cigarettes. At last he lay down and dropped rapidly through the sleep stages to stage 4 sleep, where he remained until he awoke on his own 52 minutes later. After that, he never went back to sleep at night. In short, Mr. A. slept very little except for one bout of very deep sleep. People who are sleep-deprived often have an abnormally high proportion of deep sleep, and perhaps that was what happened in Mr. A.'s case. But the worst part was his awakening for the rest of the night after less than an hour of sleep. Something about Mr. A. simply would not let him rest.

Performance tests showed just how badly Mr. A. was suffering from his inability to get restorative sleep. A Continuous Performance Test, used to measure his attentiveness, showed a score of 40 percent correct on two different days. Normally, people score between 66 percent and 78 percent correct responses during 5- or 10-minute sessions. But Mr. A.'s 40 percent was in the range for deeply sleepy people. A card-dealing exercise took Mr. A. 44 seconds, contrasted with a normal range of 15 to 26 seconds, and sorting cards into four suits required 160 seconds, as opposed to a normal range of 18 to 40 seconds.

Mr. A.'s agitated condition made some physiological tests impossible, but his doctor was able to determine, from X-ray scans and other examinations, that Mr. A. had some significant medical problems besides his insomnia, such as chronic lung disease from his continuous smoking.

An X-ray scan of his brain revealed two abnormalities. The first was a widening of the fourth ventricle, a small cavity between the cerebellum (little brain) and the pons (bridge) of the brain. This enlarged cavity is right in the area of the raphe nuclei, which helps regulate deep sleep. One might guess that the enlargement encroached on the pons structures and thus on the function of the raphe nuclei. But his doctor could not deduce the problem exactly. Future technological advances might one day uncover the mechanisms for Mr. A.'s grave sleep abnormality. For the moment, however, all that can be said is that the brain-scan finding might be related to Mr. A.'s lack of sleep, because his problem was so extreme that something was probably wrong with his sleep-regulating mechanisms.

The brain scan indicated another problem too. The frontal lobes at the very front of his brain were considerably shrunken. This brain area is much more developed in humans than in most other species and probably is responsible for some peculiarly human traits, including the ability to sit still and to inhibit our urges and curiosity. (This is one reason children have more trouble sitting still than adults do; the child's frontal lobes are not yet fully developed.) This finding from the brain scan seemed to tie in with Mr. A.'s constant agitation, his pacing around the room, and his long nightly walks. He apparently had trouble controlling himself. Moreover, with his inhibition mechanisms impaired, he was doubly affected, because his severe sleeplessness left him unable to focus his attention and concentrate on any one task for very long.

To cope with his many problems, Mr. A.'s doctor tried a variety of treatments. He administered a huge amount of diazepam (Valium), a sedative. Mr. A. was given about double a normal week's supply, administered in several doses between 8:00 P.M. and midnight, with no effect. The many prescribed drugs that Mr. A. had taken had various effects on the neurotransmitter substances that affect sleep, and none of them had worked. But there remained an important neurotransmitter, acetylcholine, whose actions could be decreased by the drugs, but not increased in any way that would be effective long term. Increasing acetylcholine can make people more alert. So Mr. A. was given an intravenous dose of a drug that briefly increases acetylcholine levels in the brain.

Acetylcholine is part of a mechanism that governs the pattern of a night's sleep. Certain nerve cells in the deep, sleep-regulating structures of the brain use acetylcholine as their neurotransmitter. When these cells spontaneously increase their electrical activity periodically during the night, deep or medium sleep is changed to REM sleep. When physostigmine, the acetylcholine-increasing drug given to Mr. A., is infused in a patient during those same states of non-REM sleep, sleep also turns to REM. When the drug is infused during REM sleep, the person awakens. Thus, physostigmine acts to alert the individual. If this drug enabled Mr. A. to become alert enough to control his behavior, a lack of acetylcholine action probably lay behind his daytime problems and possibly his sleep problems. However, an infusion of the drug made him sweat, slowed his heart rate, and raised his blood pressure, but gave him no relief from his agitation and lack of concentration.

There was still another neurotransmitter system to test with specific drugs, namely the system related to opiates. The body makes its own opiumlike neurotransmitters, the endorphins, which act on alertness as well as on mood and on perception of pain. Although Mr. A. said heroin, an opiate, had relieved his sleep problem for years, he could not be treated with this illicit drug. Morphine, however, is another opiate that is available for legitimate medical uses, and it was tried.

A small dose of morphine gave Mr. A. sound, refreshing sleep. This sudden relief after repeated failure was amazing. The drug had to be given at the right time, however—about 4:00 A.M.—to provide Mr. A. with enough refreshing sleep. This showed the pervasive influence of the biological clocks on the body—they had to be set in the right way for this small dose of drug to work. But exactly why morphine worked was anybody's guess. Some of the cells involved in regulating sleep, for example, those of the locus coeruleus, have receptor sites on their surfaces upon which opiate drug molecules can act. But they also have many other receptor sites, so it is unclear how opiates relieved Mr. A.'s insomnia from that fact alone. Much more experimentation might have been done to outline the mechanisms by which opiates helped him. For example, various cerebrospinal fluid levels of neurotransmitters could have been assayed before and after the opiates were given, and new radioactive scanning techniques could have been used to outline neurotransmitter actions or metabolic rates in various parts of his brain. But practical difficulties hinder learning; the tests involve some risk and considerable expense.

Mr. A. was released from the hospital and told to take a low dose of hydromorphone (Dilaudid), an opiate that comes in tablet form, every other night. Taking the pill in a low dose every other night would prevent habituation to the opiate and thus prevent treatment failure. This treatment worked well. Mr. A. was able to sleep about four hours every other night. This represented a huge improvement in his condition, and although it surely seems like a tiny amount to most people, it apparently was just right for Mr. A. Any more sleep, he said, caused an unpleasant feeling that he described as "speeding."

In any case, Mr. A.'s life was transformed. He put his affairs back in order, settled old debts, and acquired part interest in a service station. His appearance also improved dramatically. On follow-up visits to his doctors, he was well dressed and well groomed, remained in his seat for entire 30-minute interviews (a marked change from his former constant pacing), and was scrupulous about keeping up with his prescriptions. On his wakeful nights, he did not resort to heroin, but instead channeled his energies into productive activity, such as cleaning his service station or fixing cars. His family even welcomed him back after years of estrangement.

If he had not shown such improvement, Mr. A. could not have been treated with opiates. Permission had to be obtained from the Drug Enforcement Administration to treat him with hydromorphone; pharmacies could thereby continue to fill a prescription that otherwise might imply drug maintenance for opiate withdrawal. (A special license is needed to make this treatment available to drug addicts. Even so, some doctors, reacting to the opiate addiction in this country, are uncomfortable with or even scandalized by Mr. A.'s treatment.) Although Mr. A. required opiates, he neither progressively increased the dosage nor pressured his doctor to prescribe more than the maintenance levels of his medication. Nor did he devote increasing amounts of his life to drug taking as an addict would. In fact, he lessened his talk about drug and sleep problems, now that they were behind him, and pursued his work and family interests. By continuing to work well and to stick to the low dosage, Mr. A. showed that he was not a drug addict.

Mr. A.'s condition remains mysterious, even years later. He

had some specific disorder that began in childhood—characterized by extremely short total daily sleep time, the ineffectiveness of sedatives and various neurotransmitter-specified drugs, and ultimately successful treatment with opiates. His problem has not been diagnosed precisely and therefore was merely dropped into the general category of childhood-onset insomnia.

CHILDHOOD-ONSET INSOMNIA TREATED WITH AN ANTIDEPRESSANT

Mr. B. was a 29-year-old engineer whose childhood had been one long string of medical problems. He had suffered from insomnia since age four and was a bedwetter until he was six. He also had occasional trouble with sleepwalking, and as a child contracted a severe case of measles and an equally severe case of mumps, both accompanied by high fever. By age 14, he was showing enough daytime sleepiness to interfere with his daily routine.

He was able to cope with this problem by careful scheduling of naps and classes, and in time he became an electrical engineer and achieved professional recognition early in his career. His sleep continued to deteriorate, however, and eventually he was able to sleep only three or four hours each night—sometimes not at all. Occasional nightmares also disturbed him. Psychotherapy, relaxation exercises, and sleep-hygiene routines failed to help. At last his daytime sleepiness left him unable to work, and he received a disability pension.

Mr. B. kept a sleep log for a month and recorded bedtimes ranging from 2:30 to 3:00 A.M., with awakening between 6:00 A.M. and 7:00 A.M.—a grand total of three to four and a half hours sleep. On five nights during that month, he did not go to bed at all, and only one morning did he "sleep late" to 8:30 A.M.

He suffered from increasing depression and crying spells, and began to entertain thoughts of suicide. Under his doctors' guidance, he tried many different sedative and antidepressant drugs, none of which relieved him and some of which caused him trembling, sweating, weight loss, and even auditory hallucinations. At last, a daily 900 mg dose of lithium relieved his crying spells and self-destructive moods. (Lithium alleviates some mood disorders.)

But the basic problem, Mr. B.'s insomnia, remained unaffected. To deal with it, Mr. B. first went off drugs completely for a month, then was admitted to a hospital. An examination showed him to be depressed but otherwise normal, except for his inability to sleep at night. Nurses observing him at half-hour intervals recorded he slept 17 hours in 144 hours of observation. A nighttime polygraph made during the three and a half hours he was most likely to sleep showed he was wakeful 30 percent of the time. He had mostly medium sleep (stage 2) and REM sleep, but practically no deep sleep. This was the opposite of Mr. A., who had all deep sleep and no REM sleep. Mr. B.'s Continuous Performance Test scores ranged from 20 percent to 45 percent. Psychological tests revealed he was slightly more vulnerable to depression and anxiety than the average person, but he was remarkably strong, in view of his debilitating insomnia.

But was depression really Mr. B.'s problem? His mood but not his sleep had improved on the lithium, and his psychometric test scores did not fit the pattern of a depressive person. His sleep problem was so severe and had lasted so long that the doctor thought some other explanation was necessary.

A clue to Mr. B.'s problem turned up in an analysis of his cerebrospinal fluid. He showed low levels of serotonin metabolites. (As mentioned in chapter 1, serotonin is a neurotransmitter that regulates sleep.) A further test indicated he was not producing serotonin at a normal rate. Nothing else in his cerebrospinal fluid seemed unusual, so his doctors assumed that a relatively low serotonin output was connected with Mr. B.'s insomnia.

His doctor prescribed for Mr. B. 200 milligrams a day of trazodone (Desyrel), a drug that increases the actions of serotonin. This treatment worked; Mr. B. achieved six-hour-long spells of regular, refreshing sleep and was troubled no longer by daytime sleepiness and other disturbing symptoms. Better still, the drug had no side effects.

His insomnia relieved, Mr. B. went into a doctoral program in psychology. He chose that field because he believed it would permit him a flexible work schedule in case his sleep difficulty recurred. It did not recur, and Mr. B. became an energetic and active man. Sometimes fatigue interfered with his schoolwork, especially when he lowered his dose of trazodone, but he managed to continue his studies. He operated a psychotherapy group for disabled people, developed a busy social life, and got married.

Childhood-onset insomnia suggests an exceptional problem, because insomnia is vastly rarer in childhood than adulthood, and it suggests a disorder of greater-than-usual severity, because it disrupts the normally good sleep of the younger years. The neurological signs plus the consistency of the problem points to some structural or biochemical cause rather than to a response to life events, since most children with even major distresses in life tend to sleep well.

But beyond these generalizations, childhood-onset insomnia problems cannot be grouped together. As discussed in the case studies, radically different patterns and processes may underlie the sleeplessness. The vast range of insomnia causes—biological clock problems, nerve-cell sensitivity abnormalities, structural abnormalities, or functional impairments of different areas of the nervous system—may all theoretically contribute to childhood-onset insomnia. As varied as all these causes might be, childhood-onset insomnia does tend to be more tenacious and perplexing, on the average, than adult insomnia, and therefore seems worth considering in a special category. Perhaps sleep specialists will know better how to categorize this puzzling, apparent catchall of disorders whose common symptom is insomnia in the early years.

10
....

Other Sleep Disturbances

The roots of sleep disorders are numerous and varied, and almost any problem may damage the quality of sleep. Sleep disturbances may serve as markers of more basic medical problems that otherwise might go undetected.

Several "automatic" behavior patterns occur in the middle of sleep. They are called automatic because they do not change much, nor do they respond to environmental conditions. The sleeper continues these patterns in a basically predictable manner. For example, a sleeper may walk during sleep, sit up, wet the bed, mumble or cry out, or make chewing motions. These patterns tend to be repetitive, and poorly developed, and do not resemble the walking, sitting up, or mumbling sounds of someone who is wide awake. During sleep, however, these actions are automatic and out of context, and occur in an undisciplined way, like caricatures of normal behavior.

Such behavior occurs most often during the deepest portion of a night's sleep, during stages 3 and 4 sleep, which usually appear within the first hour after sleep begins. All of these complex automatic behaviors—complex as compared with simple behaviors such as twitching and snoring—occur much more frequently during these deep-sleep stages, possibly because the neocortex, which acts largely to inhibit behavior, does not function nearly as much during deep sleep.

These troublesome behaviors all seem to be complex sequences that are "hardwired" into a person's behavioral repertoires. They are controlled at a reflex level; no thought is necessary to chew or walk. These things are all done without conscious direction on the person's part. These patterns—urinating, sucking, and swallowing—are not suppressed during early childhood when neocortex function has not matured. Therefore, babies wet their beds. The same is true for adults who have impairments in neocortex function, such as occurs in dementia.

For unknown reasons, some people suppress some automatic behaviors less during deep sleep. Not only do the cortex-suppression mechanisms work less well, but it could be that the automatic patterns impose themselves more vehemently.

SLEEPWALKING

Sleepwalking is a behavior in which a person will arise from bed while fast asleep and walk around for a while as if awake, then return to bed. Each episode generally shows the same basic pattern of behavior. Although the sleepwalker may go through the motions of wakeful activity, he or she actually accomplishes nothing purposeful.

The entertainment industry has had a field day with sleepwalking. Comedians have seen endless opportunities to have fun with it, but there is nothing humorous about frequent sleepwalking. Many patients feel out of control and embarrassed by reports about their sleepwalking. Although the accompanying behaviors are usually harmless, the potential for problems is always present. Sleepwalkers can suffer serious falls or walk outside into the dangerous night.

Sleepwalkers apparently have some sensory mechanism working, because they do not often walk into walls, and they do perform some complex tasks, such as starting the car or filling a pan with water. The sequencing of their behavior does not add up to productive work, however; the car goes nowhere, and the pan is left on the counter. The sleepwalker is curiously unresponsive to family members who attempt to talk with him or her. The sleepwalker's eyes stare. He or she proceeds at a measured, unmodified pace and remembers nothing of the event after waking up. The sleepwalker's family finds the behavior hard to deal with; they realize that during these episodes the sleepwalker is in deep sleep.

Sleepwalking can be treated successfully. The following case history shows how giving up a stimulant can relieve a case of sleepwalking.

Ms. B., a divorced woman in her forties, had been puzzled for some time about the arrangement of pots and pans she would find in the kitchen in the morning. But she could not recall rearranging them herself, nor did anyone else in the house appear to have done it. The mystery was resolved one night when her son was awakened by a noise from the living room and found his mother sleepwalking there, unaware of her surroundings.

Ms. B. went to a sleep clinic, where she revealed she had walked in her sleep occasionally between ages seven and nine. Sometimes she had even walked to a neighbor's house. Now her sleepwalking episodes were recurring. But why?

In recent years, her life had been unusually stressful, and her sleep quality had suffered. She had had a hysterectomy six years earlier and since then had not slept as soundly as before. Before the hysterectomy, her husband had left her for another woman after 23 years of marriage. Understandably, she had experienced a certain amount of anguish in her life.

Even this, however, did not seem sufficient to explain Ms. B.'s sleepwalking. Then Ms. B. revealed her use of caffeine. She drank no fewer than 15 cups of coffee daily and sipped iced tea constantly during the summer. Her caffeine intake, combined with her recent emotional distress, appeared to be sending Ms. B. off on nocturnal rambles. She was advised to stop all caffeine. She did so, and her sleepwalking problem disappeared completely and never returned. Discontinuing drugs does not remedy every sleepwalking case, but measures to improve sleep quality are usually the first steps of effective treatment.

NIGHTMARES AND BAD DREAMS

Nightmares occur during REM sleep—and therefore later in the night—and have unpleasant emotional components such as intense fear or a feeling of being overwhelmed, threatened, or drowned. Nightmares differ from night terrors, which occur in stage 4 sleep earlier in the night and involve overwhelming emotions, panic, maximal heart rates, sweating, and other physical manifestations of emotional arousal. After a night terror, a person generally remembers very little or nothing about it. Nightmares, by contrast, tend to be highly visual experiences, although there may be auditory and tactile sensations as well; after awakening from a nightmare, a person usually recalls quite a few details. Virtually everyone has nightmares on occasion, especially during childhood. Night terrors are rarer.

Many nightmares involve themes of danger, such as being chased, beaten, drowned, confined, or about to be killed. The imagery of such dreams may be gruesome, full of horrible creatures, bloodshed, disfigurement, and murder. The sleeper may awaken in the middle of the nightmare or may sleep all the way through it, awakening the next morning with only a vague recollection of something sinister running through his or her mind.

Many nightmares are triggered by experiences that happened during the day. Unpleasant daytime events combine with the distress they cause and carry over into dreams. Some people are more susceptible to nightmares than others, just as some people are more emotional than others. One person may experience nightmares after only mildly unpleasant experiences, such as disappointments or slights, whereas someone else might require far more serious distresses.

Horribly traumatic scenes can also generate nightmares or night terrors. For instance, someone who sees a loved one die in an accident or endures a combat horror can respond with night terrors. In extreme cases, a horrible experience may continue to disturb a person's sleep for months or years afterward. Since other people can suffer such unspeakable experiences and have neither bad dreams nor night terrors, one's unique sensitivity must be provoked by the trauma. Nightmares and night terrors seem to be different processes, either of which can be triggered by emotions.

On the other hand, nightmares may not result directly from daytime experience. Psychotherapy, intended to help the patient deal with painful experiences, may also cause nightmares or bad dreams by dredging up hurtful events from the past and setting them loose in dreams. Under ordinary circumstances, a tortured memory may remain so deeply buried in a person's mind that it causes no difficulty in sleeping, but when psychotherapy brings back that memory, it can return to play havoc with the patient's sleep.

Drugs may also induce bad dreams and nightmares. Ordinary medications such as antihypertensives and steroids, both of which affect the actions of neurotransmitters in the nervous system, can cause bad dreams. Neurotransmitters play an important role in regulating emotions. Some people suffer nightmares or bad dreams, depression, headaches, or fatigue if they take drugs that affect the actions of neurotransmitters. Drugs that have effects on the body's neuroelectric systems, like those taken for heart-rhythm disturbances, may also cause bad dreams. Frightening dreams may also result from drug withdrawal, especially from stimulants, sedatives, or anticonvulsants. Depression is another major cause of bad dreams and nightmares, which can serve to warn of depression. This is one occasion when a sleep disorder may point to a much more serious underlying problem.

One case in point is that of a 35-year-old woman who was a graduate student in psychology and had horribly bad dreams. She also had a family history of depression and alcoholism, and psychotherapy had shown her how the emotional neglect she suffered in childhood had left her feeling that she must have been an unworthy individual. Psychometric tests revealed her intense depression, but sleep-laboratory records showed nothing abnormal. Assays of her blood plasma showed low levels of the amino acids tyrosine and tryptophan, building blocks for neurotransmitters. These amino acids are in our diets, but supplementing them in her diet did not help as much as she had hoped, probably because the many essential amino acids obtained from dietary protein must be transported into the nervous system by mechanisms that can only transport a limited amount of amino acids at a time. In addition, some of that capacity is used to carry other amino acids besides the ones from which neurotransmitters are made.

She tried antidepressants, but they had severe side effects, making her sweat and making her heart race when she exercised. She also took a drug to reduce her heart rate, but the drug worsened her depression. Then she tried a more specific antidepressant, trazodone (Desyrel), which affects fewer substances in the nervous system than many other antidepressants. On trazodone, her depression and bad dreams vanished without any side effects from the drug. As long as she stayed on the drug, her bad dreams remained at bay. They returned only on occasions when she ceased taking her prescription.

Every few years, her doctor tried to wean her away from the medication, but the bad dreams would reappear. Finally she withdrew from the medication and was free of bad dreams for about two years, when suddenly they returned.

There was no apparent reason for the bad dreams to reappear. Her life was going better than ever before. The doctor tried another antidepressant with few side effects, buproprion (Welbutrin), but it was ineffective, whereas trazodone helped when she resumed taking it. It seemed as if her bad dreams stemmed from something that could be relieved only by trazodone. Here, as in many other cases, doctors seemed able to relieve a symptom, but were left perplexed about why only one specific medication helped.

There is no surefire way to discover whether a person's nightmares and bad dreams are due to some largely physical cause, such as endogenous depression or the effects of medication, or whether they have mainly psychological origins. Only careful attention to the patient's history and the results of trial and error using various treatments will eventually suggest the cause. Even then, as in the graduate student described above, there remains some uncertainty. When psychotherapy provokes bad dreams, they can be used as Freud's "royal road to the unconscious" and reveal much hidden from the patient's conscious self.

Psychologically, there are quite a few ways to attempt to remedy bad dreams. Sometimes the sufferer confronts the dream, or a symbol of it, directly. The dreamer may envision a machine gun in his or her hands and use it to destroy the offending monster or whatever else plagues the dream. Some sufferers have visualized themselves surrounded by dikes that hold back rising floodwaters that symbolize overwhelming threats. Yet such approaches repress rather than solve the fundamental forces that create bad dreams. The troublesome emotions remain and are free to reemerge and cause further difficulty later.

Another, and possibly more productive, method is to try to figure out the meaning of the dreams. Sigmund Freud's pioneering work in psychotherapy uncovered in patients' dreams the remnants of thoughts and feelings from the dreamer's waking life. These remnants came mainly from recent events, notably those with emotional significance. These are mixed in with long-term feelings carried around since childhood, particularly concerning problems that had been neglected, to remain unresolved.

No one wishes to face these troublesome thoughts and feelings consciously, so in dreams they represent themselves in disguised forms that are difficult to interpret. Suppose, for example, that during childhood a boy was in constant fear of someone—a father or old brother—who was much stronger and was forever hurting him. His dreams might recall a situation where he was hurt and helpless, while his torturer was disguised as a wild animal, a monster, or some person other than the hurtful older brother or angry father. The disguise might extend still further, depending on how upsetting his conscious mind found the memory of being brutalized. Thus the dreamer might be disguised as someone else who is being hurt.

Strange combinations of present and past problems may be represented in dreams. For instance, the appearance of a new colleague at work may bring back memories of problems suffered during childhood when a new sibling appeared. On the conscious level, this connection might seem too irrational, minor, or fearsome to consider, so that old worries about competition might remain buried on the unconscious level. Yet at night, the current and former sense of threat could emerge in a dream about being menaced, displaced, or injured. Instead of the new colleague or the new sibling, a monster or threatening flood might appear. A well-known dream symbol, the house as a symbol for mother, for example, might turn up as a way of disguising the inadmissible fear that one's mother might have favored some other child in the family.

Unlike the events themselves, the unpleasant feelings that accompany them may not be disguised so easily. Indeed, dreams can amplify the terror of waking life many times over, and become as intense as the feelings we all had to suffer in the helplessness of childhood.

Even among people exposed to shocking brutality, such as the inmates of concentration camps or soldiers in battle, some will be relatively untroubled by bad dreams, while others will suffer greatly. Why? Possibly because the details of their experiences differ. More likely, however, is that some people are more vulnerable to severe distress and emotional damage than others.

Freud believed that if people were allowed to talk at length, without interruption, about whatever entered their minds, then eventually unresolved feelings would emerge on the conscious level and could be addressed. Using patients' own descriptions of their inner feelings, Freud was able to analyze and explain their dreams.

Currently, those who study dreams come from many different schools and perspectives. Some researchers and other specialists have devoted themselves to the study of dreams, from the way dreams are induced by brain lesions, daytime noise, watching movies, or wearing eyeglasses with reversing prisms, to the dream content of people of different ages, sexes, and occupations. Psychotherapists can agree on no standardized way to use dreams in therapy, but they often concur that dreams can be a valid indication of the emotional state of a person and of his or her thoughts.

More recently, some psychotherapists have used their expertise to investigate how a patient can bring hidden feelings carefully back into consciousness, in order to understand those feelings and put them behind for good. Instead of attempting to overcome and suppress the perceived dangers of the dream, the patient is encouraged to control the situation sufficiently by asking a dream figure—a monster, for example—what it "wants" or is doing there. Alternatively, the sleeper may be able to ask someone inserted purposely in the dream what is happening in the dream—why snakes or other frightening images appear there, or why he or she is being chased. The dreamer may then be able to take an answer back to the psychotherapist and discuss further the source of the troubled feelings behind the dream.

Severe nightmares and night terrors cannot be so treated because the intensity of the experiences precludes such deliberate control. Nightmares and night terrors that are a response to sudden horrible traumas often subside on their own. If they do not, daytime psychotherapy may help the person come to terms with the trauma. Childhood nightmares and night terrors are often temporary as well. But chronic bad dreams and nightmares in adults often suggest severe depression, electrical disturbance of the nervous system, drug side effects, or other ailments, and must be relieved by pinpointing their basic cause.

MOVEMENT DISORDERS

Many people lose sleep because they twitch or move constantly. One such problem is called the restless legs syndrome. This consists of agitation in the legs, twitches, and small leg movements. The sensation may rise as far as the abdomen. Mild pain and cramps may occur, sometimes with a sensation of crawling flesh shortly after bedtime. Restless legs syndrome makes the person feel an irresistible need to stand up and walk around, thus disturbing sleep. Symptoms vanish as soon as the patient stands up, then recur as soon as he or she lies down again, so that the person has a choice between no symptoms and no sleep, or considerably disturbed, damaged sleep. Eventually, the patient does fall asleep for a few hours.

Restless legs syndrome arises from conditions that affect nerves in the limbs. Diabetes may affect peripheral nerves. Disk disease affects nerves by pinching the area close to where the nerves leave the spinal cord en route to the legs. Use of diuretics is another common cause of restless legs. Normal neural electrical function depends on the presence of sodium and potassium, whose levels the diuretics alter. Furthermore, diuretics contract blood volume, which may aggravate circulation problems in the legs.

Another movement disorder is *nocturnal myoclonus,* which means "muscle twitching at night." This condition involves discrete twitches, usually in the legs, often occurring periodically every 20 to 30 seconds for long periods at night. These episodes may cause lightened sleep or may even awaken the sleeper, although they may occur without affecting sleep at all. The person's bed partner may actually notice the twitching before the person with myoclonus does. It is not known exactly what causes nocturnal myoclonus, but it may be provoked by stimulant or antidepressant medication. It is also more common in old age and in conjunction with diabetes.

Treatment of nocturnal myoclonus depends mainly on fostering good-quality sleep through sleep-hygiene methods (see chap. 11). With improved sleep quality, the individual sleeps through the frequent twitches. When medication causes the problem, as in drug side effects, the medication is changed, taken earlier in the day, or lowered in dose. Muscle-relaxing drugs such as diazepam (Valium) or baclofen (Lioresal) are frequently prescribed for nocturnal myoclonus, but infrequently relieve it. L-dopa, a drug used to control Parkinson's disease, may help in some cases.

OTHER DISORDERS OF THE BODY

Almost any physical illness worsens sleep. Usually the illness's symptoms, such as pain, itch, frequent urination, or shortness of breath, interfere with sleep. Sometimes direct physiological effects of glandular or neurological problems worsen sleep. An illness can raise or lower levels of hormones that affect good sleep (such as thyroid or steroid hormones) or interfere with normal sleep-making mechanisms (such as disturbances of neocortex function due to fever, the presence of toxins, or nerve-cell degeneration disorders). But sometimes treatment of the disease itself can make matters worse. Examples include the rash and muscle soreness following physiotherapy; the side effects of drugs that alter neurotransmitter function in the nervous system, such as thyroid hormone; nasal decongestants or antidepressants; or the scheduling difficulties of people who are attached to kidney dialysis machines two or three times a week, sometimes during night hours.

There are other ways in which illness may cause poor sleep. Sleep is likely to be impaired when a person is hospitalized. The hospital environment, with its noise, nighttime interruption for medication and monitoring, and continued crises, hardly encourages rest. And the more intensive the medical care, the worse one sleeps. According to research reports, patients in intensive care units are interrupted on average about five times per hour during the calmest periods of the night, and open-heart-surgery patients may sleep only four hours or less on the first post-operative day, when they most need rest.

A person with chronic illness may suffer a double blow where sleep is concerned, for sleeplessness itself can make some illnesses worse. Excitability at all levels of the nervous system can emerge after sleeplessness. Some people are hardly affected by a night of sleeplessness, at least in ways that psychologists can measure. But others are impatient, irritable, or depressed. In addition to decreased abilities, some functions of the nervous system may become inappropriately overactive. After two or three nights of sleeplessness—or less in many people—excessive sweating, irregular heart rhythm, nausea and vomiting, or even hallucinations can occur. Any ailment that already has such symptoms can be worsened, precipitating significant heart rhythm disturbances or seizure disorders.

Sound sleep aids recovery from illness. Good rest is indeed one of the oldest medical treatments. A dilemma arises when treatment interferes with rest. All the doctor and patient can do then is strike a balance between necessary rest and the amount of interruption that a sick person can tolerate.

A summary follows of additional sleep problems connected with illness.

Musculoskeletal disorders. Inflammation of major joints such as the hip or shoulder may make sleep difficult. The arthritic person may awaken in pain after rolling over and upsetting an inflamed joint. Ironically, painkillers used by arthritis sufferers may interfere with sleep too. So may lower-back pain when a patient suffers from diseases of the disks and must lie on his or her stomach. Back pain from ligament strains or tears may be unavoidable if the sleeper lies in a position that pulls on the tears.

Asthma. Few things are more frightening than waking up in the middle of the night with an asthma attack, fighting to breathe. The fear of such attacks alone can rob a person of sleep. So can antiasthma medications, which often have stimulant side effects.

Digestive disorders. Peptic ulcer pain can keep a person awake nights, although pain is generally worse in the daytime, provoked by meals and aggravation. But *esophagitis,* an inflammation of the esophagus causing "heartburn," is worsened by lying down. In this position, stomach acid may then seep out into the lower esophagus, where it irritates and triggers a reflex that wakes the sleeper, possibly to make him or her sit up and thus drain the acid.

Heart trouble. The pain of *angina*—a condition in which the heart muscle aches because it is not getting enough oxygen through its own blood vessels—can disturb sleep. On the other hand, sleep may protect against angina, a condition that usually seems to accompany exercise. In dreaming sleep, however, heart rate and blood pressure vary much more than in nondreaming sleep. In a patient with coronary artery disease, these cardio-vascular fluctuations result in anginal pain. Awakening with any kind of chest pain can be upsetting to the heart patient. *Prolapsed mitral valve syndrome* is a condition in which a heart-valve abnormality is accompanied by a greater sensitivity to one's own adrenalinelike neurotransmitters. This can cause insomnia, interrupted sleep, and even panic attacks at night, especially during dreams when action of these substances increases.

Itching. Of all the information a person's sensory system receives about the environment, the eyes evaluate four-fifths of it. Lying in darkness with eyes closed, people are usually much more aware of other, nonvisual senses and may be disturbed by itching that might go unnoticed during the daytime. Take away all visual distractions and itchy skin or other discomforts, such as hemorrhoids, can ruin sleep. The itch must therefore be treated with emollients, medication specific to its cause, or, in some cases, removal of an allergy-causing substance.

Kidney and liver disorders. The kidneys and liver help remove toxins from the body. But when these organs do not function properly, poisons can build up in the body and interfere with sleep. Chronic *uremia*—an accumulation of urea in the body caused by malfunctioning kidneys—may make a person insomniac. So can the dialysis treatment that is usually needed to treat uremia. Kidney dialysis treatment can disturb sleep when it is given at nighttime, or if it leaves the person extremely fatigued and prone to naps, causing maladjustments of the sleep/wake cycle. Uremic toxins can interfere with functioning of the nervous system, lowering sleep quality. Furthermore, nighttime twitching, probably due to disorders of the nervous system, is also more common in uremia.

When the liver falters or fails, insomnia may also result. Ordinarily, the liver filters out those amino acids from proteins we eat that should not be absorbed into the blood. In liver disease, however, the abnormal amino acids may not be filtered out and may pass through the liver into the circulatory system. They can get through the blood-brain barrier, limiting the entry of normal amino acids (from which normal neurotransmitters are usually made). They also can enter the metabolic pathways usually devoted to normal amino acids and may themselves be transformed into abnormal neurotransmitters. This upsets the sleep-regulating mechanisms, and the result is poor-quality sleep. Other metabolic byproducts such as ammonia, normally handled by the liver, also poison the nervous system, damaging sleep.

Epilepsy. Epilepsy patients have twice the normal prevalence of insomnia. They tend to have light sleep and some are prone to sleepwalking and night terrors. These may be triggered by abnormal brain electrical activity. Epilepsy is a generic term for a multitude of disturbances in which the brain's nerve cells have an intermittent tendency to fire too much, transmitting too many electrical impulses to neighboring nerve cells. The brain has a huge number of structures; epilepsy can affect any of them, and the symptoms that result vary accordingly. How epilepsy worsens sleep in any particular individual, however, is not known.

Menopause. Women tend to have more trouble with insomnia when they reach menopause. Fitful sleep and waking up too early in the morning are the common complaints.

Studies of these women reveal that wakeful episodes and hot flashes often begin simultaneously during sleep, as if caused by some automatic signal rather than one being caused by the other. Furthermore, studies on the disappearance of menopausal symptoms after a woman takes estrogen also show that hot flashes and sweating episodes disappear immediately. However, psychological disturbances such as depression, being unable to concentrate, or troubled sleep disappear gradually over a longer period of time.

For the average woman reaching menopause, estrogen replacements decrease sleep-onset time at the beginning of the night and increase REM sleep time significantly. Furthermore, some menopausal women with severe insomnia are relieved by taking estrogen replacements. Estrogen also prevents osteoporosis, a very significant cause of bone fractures and orthopedic problems in older women. The use of estrogen replacements has been controversial, however, because some doctors fear that the hormone will increase the chances of uterine cancer. Although uterine cancer is quite rare and is detectable early through Pap smears, estrogen may worsen cystic disease of the breast and can aggravate certain types of breast cancer. Currently, estrogen is administered in lower doses than previously and the doses are periodically accompanied by progesterone, a female hormone that causes shedding of the endometrium. This prevents the buildup of endometrial tissue, and, in theory, endometrial cancer. (It remains unknown if such estrogen-progesterone treatment increases the incidence of breast cancer.)

In each case, the patient and her gynecologist must weigh the risks and benefits of estrogen replacement after careful review of the patient's postmenopausal symptoms, family history of breast cancer, and risk of developing osteoporosis.

SLEEP APNEA: WHEN BREATHING STOPS

Apnea means "no breathing," and sleep apnea is a condition in which a sleeper ceases to breathe for short periods. Sleep apnea is most common in middle-age and older overweight men. Such men snore loudly and stop breathing during sleep for 10- to 60-second periods or even longer. In extreme cases, a man may stop breathing several hundred times during the night. Men with this condition tend to have short, thick necks and swollen tissues in their airways or fatty tissue at the base of their tongues. Also, the muscles at the back of the throat relax too much during sleep, so that the tongue and flaccid muscles flap around in the upper airway, causing snoring and sometimes cutting off the airway completely for a while.

About 20 percent of adults snore, and there are many overweight men in the world. But snoring and overweight do not necessarily indicate sleep apnea. The presence of *additional* symptoms, especially excessive sleepiness during the day, increase the likelihood that a person has the disorder. Many sleep-apnea patients have a hard time staying awake while seated and unoccupied for any length of time—for example, in a meeting, driving on an interstate highway, or watching a movie. Extremely loud snoring or the presence of high blood pressure also increases the likelihood of sleep apnea.

The effects of sleep apnea on general health are still unclear. Although very common, sleep apnea was discovered only about 25 years ago, probably because not much research on sleep problems was done before then and also because some people show no specific daytime signs of the condition. Although overweight men are the most common patients, they are not the only ones predisposed to the condition. Anyone with a very narrow upper airway may have sleep apnea, including children who snore because they have large adenoids and tonsils, and even some slender women with upper airway impediments, such as a slightly recessed jaw that pushes the tongue back a bit into the throat airway.

The reason sleep apnea might be much more common in men than in women (the ratio varies between about 8 to 15 male patients for every 1 female, depending on the group studied) is the greater thickness of tissues in men. Also, a female hormone, progesterone, stimulates respiration and therefore may help prevent breathing problems. Finally, many normal-weight men have repeated periods during the night when they stop breathing for 15 to 30 seconds or longer, but they still show no daytime symptoms. And some very obese men have no sleep apnea at all. Some people can tolerate a lot more disturbed sleep than others, while not even feeling it the next day. And although they may have the same level of carbon dioxide in the bloodstream—the major stimulus for breathing—some make less respiratory effort than others and are therefore more likely to stay breathless longer when something hinders their breathing. How strong the effort is to overcome a hindrance may be partly determined by hereditary factors. Those who make more effort might be the ones that remain apnea free.

Sedatives, especially alcohol, significantly impair breathing. The wives of sleep-apnea patients frequently note that their husbands snore more after having a few drinks in the evening. Tranquilizers and sleeping pills might also worsen sleep apnea.

Heart disease, lung disease, and degenerative conditions of the nervous system can predispose a person to sleep apnea. They do so by upsetting some of the physiological mechanisms that regulate breathing. A slowing of blood circulation, for example, delays vital information carried to the brain about the amount of oxygen and carbon dioxide in the blood leaving the lungs.

Lowered metabolic rate, which occurs in sleep and is common in older people in general, lessens the strength of a person's normal tendency to breathe harder when blood carbon dioxide increases. Thus blood carbon dioxide, a regular waste product of our metabolism, can increase beyond its usual levels before the apnea patient makes the breathing response that would excrete the carbon dioxide from the lungs by exhalation. During this prolonged interval before a breathing response occurs, blood oxygen level keeps falling.

If the interval, or apnea period, is long enough, blood oxygen can fall to levels low enough to trigger emergency reflexes that induce rapid breathing. But a desperately strong, sudden attempt to inspire air, intended to move it quickly to the lungs, can generate a big difference in pressure between the lungs and the outside air. The pressure can be great enough to suck the airway closed, especially an airway made flaccid and flabby from sedatives, age, illness, fatigue, or obesity. Thus, the maximal breathing effort shuts down airflow altogether.

Eventually, the reflexes lighten sleep or awaken the apnea patient, who takes a breath and rapidly falls back to sleep. But this cycle of events can occur dozens or even hundreds of times a night, disturbing sleep and making the person sleepy during the day. It is a subtle form of body torture, sometimes unfelt by the patient, who keeps needing sleep but never sleeps well because he or she breathes so poorly during it.

Chronic lung disease complicates the condition by intensifying the apnea. The lung disease prevents an efficient exchange of gases between the blood and the inhaled air, causing carbon dioxide buildup in the blood. The tendency to breathe too hard suddenly is amplified, and apnea occurs more readily. In more severe states of lung disease, too little oxygen in the blood can provoke unusually strong inspirations that shut down the sleeper's airway.

At this point it seems that sleep apnea is a generic term for a host of problems that can interfere with breathing during sleep.

Sleep apnea can have dire consequences. The patient never sleeps long enough at a stretch to obtain good-quality sleep, so he or she is always sleepy during the day. Moreover, the patient does not remember why he or she was unable to sleep the night before, because the patient never woke up completely during these short breaks in sleep. Thus, the sleep apnea sufferer stumbles through the next day's activities in a groggy condition, without realizing what is wrong.

Another kind of sleep apnea is caused not by blockage of the airway during sleep but rather by some failure of the nervous system to signal the breathing muscles to keep moving. This kind of sleep apnea also makes its sufferers sleepy during the day, but they tend to complain more of wakefulness during the night.

Both kinds of sleep apnea are potentially serious. They are often associated with high blood pressure and sometimes with irregular heart rhythms, because the heart tries to work harder during the apnea episodes and can become enlarged. Moreover, sleepy people are susceptible to accidents, which may be the worst health hazard of sleep apnea. Sleep apnea requires the specialized facilities of a sleep laboratory and clinic to diagnose it reliably and treat it promptly.

SLEEP APNEA TREATMENT

C-PAP is short for *continuous positive airway pressure,* a method of treating snoring and sleep apnea. To help breathing during sleep, a mask over the sleeper's face provides air at slightly increased pressure, which allows easier breathing. (There are home health-care companies that will bring the small C-PAP machine to a patient's home and, under supervision, work with the patient to make the C-PAP comfortable and effective.) The added "push" on the air helps the "pull" of the patient's diaphragm and chest muscles. Airway structures are widened, and air flows more easily. As a result, muscles lining the airway and structures such as the soft palate are no longer sucked into the airstream where they vibrate noisily and impede airflow. The sleep-apnea patient's snoring ceases. So do the periods of failed breathing and the continual brief spells of wakefulness. At last the patient has a good night's sleep, and his or her daytime functions improve greatly.

Sleep apnea can be relieved, in many cases, by a fairly new surgical technique sometimes called uvulopalatopharyngo-plasty. This is surgical jargon for revision of the uvula, the structure hanging down from the soft palate in the midline of the throat. The operation also involves revision of the palate and tightening up of the throat's lining. About half of patients with sleep apnea also have nasal abnormalities, such as a deviated septum or other structures that are enlarged and partially block their nasal passageways. Blockage of the passageways is worse when a person lies down, because gravity no longer helps drain the thickened tissues. Nasal surgery to correct the blockage is often done at the same time as the throat surgery, so sometimes the entire procedure is called *revision of the upper airway*.

Generally speaking, surgery has the best results in the less obese patient. In one recent study of sleep-apnea sufferers who underwent upper airway surgery, the postoperative results showed dramatic improvement. One patient, a 38-year-old production supervisor, was interviewed four months after his operation and reported that it had changed his life. He was no longer weary. He couldn't take a nap during the day if he tried, and he had astonished his employers by coming up with some new business innovations. In fact, he felt so much more energetic that he had taken a second job evenings and Saturdays when he previously had been asleep. Other patients showed comparable improvements. But opinions vary sharply about how much surgery helps. The procedure was developed relatively recently. Not many ear, nose, and throat surgeons were really comfortable doing this operation at first, and many have had little experience with it, compared with others who have refined their techniques through scores of procedures.

Judging whether the operation has been a success has also been a problem. In many cases, laboratory records of an apnea patient's sleep after upper-airway revision surgery have shown little or no improvement in selected breathing measures. The patients, however, nearly all feel more awake and energetic during the day. Although sleep doctors have ascribed some patients' glowing reports to a placebo effect, such patients really fare better, according to interviews with their families or co-workers. All this suggests that sleep doctors are not measuring the real factors that make sleep-apnea patients sleep (see chap. 12).

CHANGING HABITS TO OBTAIN OPTIMUM BENEFITS FROM TREATMENT

Mr. G. wrote and sold advertising for a small magazine. During 15 years of marriage, his wife had become concerned over his snoring and what she called his "sleep cycles." These were 10- to 18-second periods in which he would cease to breathe. At the end of each period, he would take a giant breath, exhale, inhale and exhale again four or five times, and then cease breathing for another 10 to 18 seconds. His wife reported that he was very restless in his sleep.

After such restless nights, Mr. G. would drag himself groggily out of bed, head aching. The ragweed season was especially hard on Mr. G. His nose stopped up, and all his other problems got worse—the snoring, the struggles during sleep, the morning headaches. During the day, Mr. G. felt sleepy. Sometimes he would fall asleep at work.

Like most sleep-apnea sufferers, Mr. G. had a serious problem with weight and overeating. While driving along New England turnpikes on business trips, he would munch on sandwiches purchased in coin machines, and wash them down with gallons of diet soda. His diet of fats and starches helped pack 280 pounds onto his five-foot-eight-inch frame. He had tried to lose weight, but like 90 percent of people who shed pounds, he put them right back on. Once he had even gone to a psychologist who advised him to see how long he could go without eating, a useless exercise. Fasting or crash diets make some people so weak that they cannot lift their heads off the pillow, and any weight lost is usually regained as soon as the person stops fasting. That was Mr. G.'s experience on a no-calorie diet.

One day a physician saw Mr. G. asleep at a party and advised him to visit a sleep clinic. In the clinic's sleep laboratory, Mr. G. stopped breathing 412 times during the night. Usually he would stop breathing for 15 to 30 seconds, slightly longer than his wife's estimate. But once he stopped breathing for 66 seconds. During these apnea spells, the oxygen saturation of the red cells in his blood would fall to half the normal value. His heart would slow down to 50 or 54 beats per minute, then would speed up suddenly to 90 or more when he breathed again. This pattern indicated stress on his heart. He got no deep sleep at all, which probably explained why he was sleepy in the daytime.

An ear, nose, and throat surgeon with much experience in treating sleep apnea examined Mr. G. and found he had some upper airway problems, including a significantly deviated nasal septum, the bone-and-cartilage "wall" that separates the nasal passages. The septum, displaced to one side, could interfere with breathing, especially when Mr. G. lay down.

Other breathing problems also afflicted Mr. G. when he was in a reclining position: it fatigued his diaphragm (the sheet of muscle just below the lungs that contracts during inspiration), because gravity could not help to move his distended belly out of the way, as it did when he stood upright. Tissue fluid tended to accumulate in his head when he lay down, too, because gravity could not help to drain it. It is tissue fluid that makes one's face puffy after a night's sleep. In Mr. G.'s case, the fluid built up in his head overnight and bloated the tissues in his airway, restricting his breathing even more.

Using a flexible fiber-optic scope that can peer deeply into the breathing passages, the surgeon also discovered a problem with the function of the soft tissue of Mr. G.'s throat. When Mr. G. breathed through his mouth while lying down, his throat tissues collapsed into his airway. But at the same time, his narrowed nose passages, partially blocked when he lay down, encouraged him to breathe through his mouth.

This daunting set of problems had not developed overnight.

They had accumulated gradually over the years, while Mr. G. grew accustomed to poor nighttime sleep and the daytime drowsiness that followed.

Mr. G. could have continued this way, but he needed relief. First, he needed to lose weight. The thinner he was, the more effective any apnea treatment would be. So he was put on a weight-loss program. It would not provide immediate relief for his breathing and sleeping problems, but it was an important step in his total treatment.

Mr. G. started by keeping a chart of everything he ate and drank, and at the time he ate or drank it. The chart showed he ate 6 to 10 times daily, usually meat or cheese on bread, plus occasional helpings of chicken or tuna salad and cookies. He believed that small carbohydrate meals stimulated him, whereas large helpings made him sleepy.

It is just this kind of continual ingestion of carbohydrates that keeps many patients' appetites overly activated. They undergo constant cycles of hunger and carbohydrate intake, which satisfies them momentarily and may even stimulate them so that they feel better for the moment. But the carbohydrates are absorbed so quickly that they boost the person's blood sugar and thus cause a rapid secretion of insulin, which in turn brings on a more rapid metabolism and causes blood sugar to fall. The drop in blood sugar makes the eater crave more carbohydrates, and the cycle starts all over again. The problem is compounded by feelings of pleasure and reward, creating conditioned reflexes that encourage further carbohydrate consumption. The result is that many overweight people continue to eat meals of sweets, starches, and baked goods that keep them fat.

Most people begin by trying to lose weight on their own. Those who remain courageous enough to bring up the problem with their doctor are often referred to a nutritionist, which is an effective way to begin. The nutritionist will most often require a written record of all food consumed and when it was eaten, like the chart Mr. G. kept. The circumstances provoking dietary slips will be examined. Analyzing the person's schedule, dietary habits, self-esteem, and fears of discouragement are all elements in a successful weight-loss program.

In order to refrain from constant intake of carbohydrates, Mr. G. was placed on a low-carbohydrate diet and his meals restricted to five a day. Out went the bread and cookies; in came chicken roll, lean roast beef, and cauliflower (his preferences). Instead of buying sandwiches while driving down the turnpike, Mr. G. took along a bowl of broccoli and raw red cabbage to munch on as needed. While awaiting his upper airway surgery, he also used C-PAP to allow easy breathing while asleep.

The results were gratifying. Mr. G. shed 60 pounds and continued to lose weight. He felt greatly relieved, and at last he got a good night's sleep. His morale soared as his daytime drowsiness disappeared. Eventually Mr. G. had the surgery, which awakened him significantly and, as it often does, gave him the energy and determination to stick with the diet. This case is not exceptional. Other patients in Mr. G.'s position actually prefer the largely vegetarian diet and could not return to the heavy foods they ate previously.

For many, the term *sleep disorder* implies insomnia. Although insomnia may be by far the most common sleep complaint, sleep quality can suffer in many other ways. Often disturbed sleep is never discovered because the sleeper never detects it, and a movement disorder during sleep or sleep apnea is first spotted by a person's spouse or other relative. Even then, a person may feel the problem is not worth investigating, a solution particularly true of sleep-apnea patients. But such people often feel vastly better when their sleep quality is improved.

11
....

What You Can
Do About Poor Sleep

The key to relieving poor sleep is an alliance between doctor and patient. Yet there are steps you can take without a doctor's help. Like the patients described in this book's case histories, you can keep a sleep chart, discontinue use of sleep-disrupting drugs, start an exercise program, and do progressive relaxation exercises. Even if self-help fails to improve your sleep, it provides a good beginning that will complement a doctor's efforts. This chapter shows you how to combine a few specific ways to improve sleep into a larger program of sleep hygiene.

SLEEP CHARTING

Keep a month-by-month record of your sleep. A sleep chart is the basic way you can document and keep track of your sleep disturbances. Using sleep charts, you can see how much your sleep improves or deteriorates as months pass and how various treatments affect your sleep. A daily record of information about your sleep will help maintain your interest as you continue with current remedies or find some better ones. It might even help maintain habits that foster good sleep and discourage those that

disrupt sleep. But for any sleep disturbance that you help manage, you will need to make a sleep chart. Even if you have a
problem that is mainly managed by the doctor, such as insomnia
due to hyperthyroidism or sleepwalking set off by antiasthma
medications, your records will help measure the success of treatment.

Make a chart with four columns: one column each for the
date, the time you turned out the light and tried to get to sleep,
the time you arose from bed, and a final column for any special
comments or observations you may have that day. You may
have felt ill, taken a sleeping pill, stayed up to watch television,
or had a tough day at work. That last column can be especially
informative. Your comments may point to something that especially harmed your sleep, such as a drink or cup of coffee in
the evening. What you keep track of in such a column depends
on your individual situation. Night classes, exercise, heavy
meals, unpleasant obligations, use of medications, number of
cigarettes smoked—anything you regularly do that somehow
affects your sleep should be charted at first. Gradually, as some
factors emerge as more relevant to sleep quality, charting can
focus on them.

After a month, you will be able to look at the record and see
how regular your bedtimes and arising times were. You will
be able to spot any connections between your sleep schedule
and the things you mentioned in the observations column on
your chart. You also may see a connection between things you
did one day and the way you felt the next day.

This is a very simple sleep chart. With a little extra effort,
you can keep a much more revealing chart. Take a pencil and
ruler and divide a sheet of paper into a matrix of 31 lines (one
for each day of the month) perpendicular to 24 lines (one for
each hour of the day). (See figs. 4–6.) Designate one line toward
the middle of the chart as 3:00 A.M., when most people are
asleep, so that your nighttime sleep period will be centered
neatly on the chart. Leave a few extra columns at the side to
note things that affect your sleep. This matrix will allow you
to keep track of your sleeping and waking hours for every hour
of the month.

The morning is a good time to chart each night's sleep, while it is fresh in your mind. For each night, make a vertical mark when you turned out the light to go to sleep, then start a horizontal line when you think you fell asleep. Keep the horizontal line solid for the times you were asleep, but interrupt it for the times you were awake. If you are constantly awake, or sleep only briefly, make a dashed line. Absolute accuracy is *not* required. In fact, you will never sleep well if you make sleep charting a full-time job. All you need from the chart is a reasonable idea of what occurred during the night. End the horizontal line when you wake up for the day, and make another vertical mark to indicate when you got out of bed. If you arise for an extended period during the night, longer than just a few minutes to go to the bathroom, mark this period with vertical lines. Be sure also to indicate naps you may take during the day.

At the end of the month, you will be able to see the regularity, or irregularity, of your sleep schedule. You can note any consistent patterns such as regular awakening at a certain hour, or any consistent tendency of your sleep schedule: for example, bedtimes, middle-of-the-night waking periods, or arising times that slide progressively later or earlier on the clock. Here again, you can see a connection between the sleep problem and factors that may affect sleep.

This matrix chart provides an instant visual readout of your sleep patterns. It is a detailed graphic and more easily comprehensible than a chart that records only clock times, because it puts the clock times in a context and reveals patterns over the course of a month. With the diagnostic information that the matrix chart provides, you can obtain an overview of your baseline sleep and judge subsequently whether any treatment you tried may actually help relieve your sleep problem.

When asked to make a sleep chart, many people say, "Oh, I know my sleep pattern: It's wake up at two in the morning and no sleep for the rest of the night," or some other perceived pattern. But the actual record itself reveals variations in sleep patterns. Individual problems may also become obvious, such as delayed sleep-phase syndrome, hyperarousal insomnia, sensitivity to caffeine, or the early waking associated with depression.

There is another, surprising benefit to this kind of sleep chart. It seems to help people sleep. Many patients who had been able to remedy their insomnia asked their sleep-clinic doctor, on their last visits, for a few sleep charts to maintain over the following months, even though they were sleeping well. And when given a sleep chart to complete, patients who had suffered relapses after sleeping well for a time slept better without further treatment.

Merely keeping a sleep chart, then, seems to offer some non-specific aid to sleep. Possibly the chart makes the person think more about his or her sleeping habits, keep a better schedule knowing that it must be recorded on the chart, and avoid sleep-disrupting influences because they too would appear on the chart. Whatever the reason, keeping a sleep chart seems to be one of the best therapies someone bothered with poor sleep can try.

SELF-HELP MEASURES

Since sleep is a general barometer of your health and daytime functioning, almost everything affects it one way or another. Most people have enough reserve and flexibility in their sleep-regulating systems to tolerate potential sleep problems like those caused by a late night or cold medication and still feel they get adequate sleep. But for those who tend to have sleep problems, a few adjustments in sleep routine give them a better chance to weather potential disturbances. Often patients ask, "Must I do all these things to improve my sleep, or might I just try one or two of them to see how they will work?" Quite simply, you are most likely to sleep well if you practice *all* the measures in this section. After you are free of sleep problems for a few months, you might discontinue some of the measures one at a time to see if you can get away with making less effort to maintain your sleep. Here again are the basic steps toward better sleep:

1. Stop using any drugs that may affect the nervous system. The major culprits are caffeine, alcohol, and tobacco. Discontinue nose drops (except saline-solution drops) and nasal decongestant pills. Modify intake of all prescribed medications that act on the nervous system if you can, but only under your physician's supervision. Ask your doctor if it is possible to substitute other drugs for any stimulating antidepressant or beta-blocker medications you might be taking; most of these drugs have to be discontinued gradually, over a month's time. Sedatives, tranquilizers, and sleeping pills may need to be tapered down over two months' time.

2. Get up at the same early hour each day, even on your days off, and no matter how well or poorly you slept the night before. This will help you avoid the late-sleeping syndrome (see chap. 3). Seven in the morning or earlier seems safe. Go out into the sunlight for approximately a half hour shortly afterward so that the bright light will help set your internal clocks. (In northern climes during the winter, try to get into outdoor light early in the day.) Avoid irregular naps, and don't stay in bed longer than you sleep.

   The actual dose of bright light and the best time of day for it has yet to be worked out. We know that regularly timed bright light early in the day helps reset the circadian rhythms for a 24-hour period. This helps prevent delays in bedtimes and arising times. Any dose and timing of light that proves effective, therefore, should be continued.

3. Keep regular mealtimes. Shift the majority of your food intake toward morning rather than evening. Have a small supper several hours before bedtime. Note from your sleep chart if a meal full of carbohydrates (foods high in flour, starches, or sugar) at supper worsens sleep.

4. Have a regular, predictable evening routine. Learn meditation procedures or muscle-relaxation exercises. After you have mastered them, practice them shortly before bedtime and during any waking periods at night. Soak

in water as hot as you can tolerate in the bathtub, with as much of your body immersed as possible, for 20 minutes in the evening—enough to increase your body temperature. Of course, take care standing up; a hot tub soak can make you feel faint if you get up too suddenly. (Caution: People with any heart problem should obtain their physician's approval before soaking in a hot tub.)

5. Make regular exercise a habit. But before beginning a regular exercise program, you should consult with your physician, particularly if you are age 35 or older. After getting a physician's clearance, you will need to exercise a minimum of three times a week—every other day— to derive benefit. The exercise must raise your heart rate to about 60 to 85 percent of your maximum for at least 20 minutes a session. (Your maximum heart rate is 220 minus your age.) You can, of course, do less strenuous exercise for longer periods. Consult a sports-medicine doctor or accredited fitness specialist. He or she can get you started on a safe, long-term program. Safe and effective exercise programs can also be developed for people with high blood pressure, heart disease, arthritis, or any other limiting condition.

6. Rid yourself of nighttime annoyances. If you must urinate frequently, train your bladder. Gradually prolong the time between your first urge to urinate and relieving yourself during the day, increasing the interval 15 minutes each week until it reaches 90 full minutes. Then drink an extra 20 ounces of water mornings, but no liquids after supper in the evening. Shed excess weight to ease back pain, snoring, and hiatus hernia pain when lying down.

Compare your sleep charts before and after taking these six steps. If none of these measures helps, see a sleep doctor. At the very least, you will have helped the doctor determine the source of your sleep problem and a course of treatment for it.

If you suspect your difficulty is endogenous depression, take measures quickly to deal with it. Have a medical or psychiatric evaluation promptly. Many people are inclined to delay doing something about depression, hoping that it will go away. They may wish to avoid talking about their personal problems or feel ashamed of their condition or fear turning into someone like a depressed co-worker or family member they dislike. Overcoming denial and procrastination is the first step toward effective treatment. Also, treatment for depression, including antidepressants, may take a long time to work, so the longer you wait, the longer relief will require. Be frank with your doctor about all the drugs you may be using, and take any of the doctor's prescriptions faithfully according to instructions.

FROM HOME REMEDIES TO L-TRYPTOPHAN

It seems that almost everyone has some pet remedy to offer for insomnia. One widely touted trick, more than a mere folk remedy, is to drink a cup of warm malted milk before going to bed. Experimental studies have shown that the milk actually does help in many cases, more than the placebo effect explains.

One investigation reported in the *British Medical Journal* in 1972 compared sleep quality after taking a hot malted milk at bedtime with sleep after swallowing an inert capsule. The researchers suggested that the pill contained a folk remedy for sleeplessness, so that everyone involved in the study, milk drinkers and pill takers alike, believed they were taking something to encourage sound sleep. On some nights, subjects took the capsule, on other nights they had malted milk instead.

Records made in the sleep lab showed that the subjects had fewer body movements on the nights they drank the milk than on nights when they took the inert capsules. The beneficial effect of malted milk was most pronounced in the latter part of the night, and grew more noticeable with continued usage over several nights. The malted milk was most effective on a group of volunteers aged 42 to 65, who averaged about 11 minutes more sleep each night. They also exhibited about 20 minutes less intervening wakefulness at night. This effect became more marked with continued use—just the opposite of what happens using hypnotic medications.

A Freudian might be attempted to draw a connection between the effects of malted milk and comforting childhood memories. But there may be another, chemical factor involved. Some sleep specialists recently have investigated an amino acid called *l-tryptophan,* which is found in milk and other foods including poultry, fish, and eggs, and is available in health-food stores in tablet form. Taken at bedtime, l-tryptophan appears to help subjects get to sleep more rapidly, but, unlike milk, it does not seem to help them return to sleep after awakening during the night. Thus, the two substances may act by different means.

The best guess of biochemists is that l-tryptophan plays some role in the production of serotonin (see chap. 1). It is also possible, however, that l-tryptophan encourages sleep by stimulating production of certain soporific hormones in the intestinal tract. The malt used in the British study may have a similar effect.

L-tryptophan used as a sleeping aid is not as powerful as synthetic drugs, but it works reliably for some people and poses some advantages over drugs. For example, l-tryptophan does not appear to interfere with normal EEG patterns, causes no side effects, and does not generate problems with tolerance and withdrawal. Like every other treatment, l-tryptophan is not a surefire cure-all for sleep disorders. Although trying l-tryptophan is not harmful, the pills are large and can be very expensive. Dr. Ernest Hartmann of Tufts Medical School found that 2 grams (four of the usual pills) provided about the maximal effect, and even 1 single gram had a significant effect.

In the final analysis, the best self-therapy is simply the one that works best for you. If l-tryptophan seems to help, or a glass of warm milk (malted or not), or eating a warm blueberry muffin, fine. Pursue that approach without overindulging in it, and you will probably benefit from it.

12
....

Professional Help

If you sleep poorly, start with self-help. You can do many things without a doctor's assistance to encourage better sleep. If self-help fails, however, then professional help may be advisable. Before entering a course of treatment, understand that doctors rarely perform instant miracles. Patients with sleep problems that have lasted for years call sleep-disorder clinics hoping to be seen and relieved within a few days. Sometimes they feel that admission to a hospital will relieve their problems. But your environment and daily routines affect your sleep profoundly. The hospital is an artificial environment far removed from normal life and therefore is not a good place to treat most sleep problems.

Professional treatment of a sleep disorder may last months or even years. Even then, relief may be elusive for a small minority of patients. There are conditions that the most capable doctor cannot correct and that the most careful diagnosis may overlook. Some clinics specialize in certain disorders and treatments, and this emphasis may work to the disadvantage of patients who have other problems. Most physicians, however, will refer a patient to an alternative source if the patient's problem does not fall into the doctor's area of expertise, and a sleep clinic generally has much to offer a person with a sleep disorder.

Many people who suffer from sleep disturbances could correct them on their own. On the other hand, many who suffer from troubled sleep try for years to cope unaided with significant medical problems, when treatment by a doctor might correct the trouble.

SHOULD YOU GO TO A SLEEP CLINIC?

In earlier chapters, we have seen a sampling of conditions that may harm sleep. A short list of questions follows. It will help you determine whether a sleep-disturbing condition is serious and intractable enough to require professional help, or whether the problem can be overcome by a change of habits.

1. *How often do you get less sleep than you think adequate?* If you suffer poor sleep more often than you would like, or feel that poor sleep quality affects you the next day, and if you have tried to remedy this without success, then a visit to a sleep clinic may be advised. The same can be said if you feel you are sleepier than everyone else around you, or worry a lot about whether you will be alert enough to deal with some scheduled event, from an evening engagement to a business meeting. A sleep clinic consultation might help.

2. *Do you have problems that occur while you are asleep?* If you suffer from various troubles during sleep, such as bad dreams, sudden awakening with paralysis or in panic, or even sleepwalking, these are worth examining at a sleep-disorder clinic. Sometimes other people, usually family members or roommates, tell the sleeper about problems that the sleeper doesn't recall: constant restlessness, thunderous snoring, or crying out. Even though a family member might suggest medical investigation, some sleepers who don't know about these symptoms often want to avoid consulting a doctor. This often happens with sleep-apnea patients, whose snoring,

high blood pressure, obesity, and/or heart problems
may worry family members more than it worries the
sufferer.

3. *Have you discussed your sleep problem with a doctor?* If you
already feel concerned enough about your sleep quality
to have mentioned it to a doctor, you probably have a
sleep problem worth investigating further. Talk to your
physician in detail.

4. *Do you use alcohol or other drugs to help induce sleep?* In-
frequent use of sleep-promoting drugs is probably
harmless. Nearly everyone takes something now and
then to help bring on sleep when unsettled matters in
daily life interfere with slumber. Frequent use of medications to induce sleep, however, is a matter for concern
and should be discussed with a doctor.

5. *Does nighttime noise or some other disturbance in your environment trouble you often?* This in itself is nothing unusual. We all must cope with sirens, aircraft noise, or
other small disturbances at night. If you have considerable trouble returning to sleep after these upsets, however, then you may have a sleep disorder that would
benefit from professional treatment.

A "yes" answer to any of these questions indicates a problem
of some significance. If practicing good sleep hygiene along
with consultation with your physician does not correct the problem, then a visit to a sleep clinic may well be advisable.

SEEKING TREATMENT

Some people know they have a problem, but do not seek help
because they have made their own diagnosis and decided their
case is hopeless. Insomnia patients, in particular, often decide
they cannot sleep because of a troublesome problem about
which they feel helpless—a boss, a troubled child, or financial
worries. Of course, worrying does not help sleep, but other
difficulties, such as sensitivity to caffeine, drug side effects, sleep

apnea, or problems with internal clocks might really be the cause of the problem.

SLEEP CLINICS

Sleep-disorders medicine is a new field full of controversy, and sleep-clinic practices vary widely. Clinics range from those that will see all types of problems and offer treatment by staff physicians, to those whose interest might be primarily in diagnosing a sleep problem while referring the patient elsewhere for treatment. The clinic might also have a specialization in only one or two types of sleep disorders. Some clinics are outgrowths of research programs and will take on the cases of only those people whose sleep problem relates to the clinic's interest, although this practice is less common now than in previous years. People are accepting more and more that sleep disorders are legitimate problems worth medical attention, and this acceptance will encourage more clinics to operate.

Treatment of sleep disorders often requires careful adjustments over a long period. The narcolepsy patient, for example, needs to work gradually toward an optimal dosage of medication and develop the best sleep and daily schedules. This requires keeping detailed records of when troublesome symptoms occur and when sound sleep is obtained. Similar long-term work is needed for most other sleep disorders.

As mentioned, sleep-disorder clinics may diagnose a sleep problem and then send the patient for treatment elsewhere. This approach is appropriate in some instances such as in sleep-apnea conditions that require surgical treatment or insomnia from depression that requires antidepressants. But many patients need long-term care from physicians experienced in the treatment of sleep disorders, and such care remains relatively difficult to find at this time.

THE SLEEP LABORATORY

Most sleep clinics put patients in the sleep laboratory for a night. A night in the laboratory costs about $700 to $1,300. Most sleep clinic costs are covered by medical insurance, but insurance companies differ in their reimbursement policies—so check your policy. Given the expense and potential importance of that one night, it should be prepared for carefully.

In the early 1970s, to obtain measurements of nighttime sleep that were not disrupted by bad daytime habits, some clinics began to require that patients structure and control their daytime hours. They were asked to give up caffeine, alcohol, and other drugs that affect the nervous system so that the laboratory could get a real rather than an amplified or distorted view of the insomnia—and therefore have a better chance of finding the insomnia's cause. Furthermore, patients had to keep a sleep chart prior to the laboratory session so that the lab could begin re-cordings when the patients' internal clocks were set for bedtime and sleep. Patients were also required to get up at a regular time daily so that they would normalize their bodies' schedules.

After following these measures for a few weeks, many patients called and explained they did not need to sleep in a lab-oratory after all; their insomnia was cured. In fact, it became evident not only that these laboratory-preparation measures helped, but that patients slept a great deal better in the sleep lab than they predicted. Dr. William Dement of Stanford University observed that patients greatly underestimated their sleep. Ironically, Dr. Dement's findings seemed to emphasize the subjective nature of insomnia and made objective confirmation of it more difficult. It became clear that there is no reliable way to measure insomnia scientifically, and in some cases it became a complaint without laboratory verification. Sleep doctors had a difficult time objectively rating how bad a patient's sleep was and whether it actually improved after treatment.

A few sleep specialists decided that the laboratory was not revealing enough about the causes of insomnia and that less emphasis should be placed on measuring sleep in a lab, and obtaining questionable results, and more effort put into other means of insomnia measurement, such as sleep charts. Some even decided that insomnia was too complex and too psychologically based, and therefore treatment was too ineffective to justify the effort. Others emphasized simple measures that seemed to help and could be applied in a systematic manner to relieve the sleep problem—whether or not their mechanisms of effect were understood.

A group of treatment measures developed around this last idea, most of which are described in this book: regular rising times, charting sleep, eliminating drugs that affect the nervous system, evening relaxation exercises, temperature-raising methods such as vigorous exercise or hot tub soaks, bright-light routines, and regular meals. These were considered nonspecific methods that all insomnia patients should begin with and came to be known as sleep hygiene. Many clinics continue to emphasize them.

But another school believed that even if the sleep laboratory did not turn up information that would benefit all patients, some important data might be discovered for some of them. Furthermore, a few of the patients might have sleep apnea or nocturnal myoclonus, serious conditions that could be diagnosed only in a laboratory. As a result, many sleep doctors are trying to find less expensive alternatives to current laboratory methods. Some are using home monitoring with small cassette recorders that monitor body temperature and movements and provide information about the sleep/wake cycle and internal clocks.

Recently, Dr. Peter Hauri of the Mayo Clinic reported that insomnia patients showing no real sleep disorders during one night in the sleep laboratory did in fact demonstrate poor sleep when they were monitored by a wrist actigraph. An actigraph simply monitors body movements. From the recorded movements it is possible to distinguish sleep from wakefulness and establish a continuous record of sleep over several days and nights. Since sleep can vary so greatly from night to night, actigraph studies may produce better information about patterns of insomnia than a single night in the laboratory. Dr. Hauri had only a small sampling of patients, but for those who would otherwise be diagnosed as having "no objective findings," he found that the sleep laboratory polygraph overestimated sleep by more than an hour per night if compared to wrist actigraph recordings. The patients' sleep was abnormally restless when measured against other groups. Unfortunately, portable recording outside the sleep laboratory is still a rarity, and there are reasons for continued use of the laboratory method. Some patients travel great distances to a sleep clinic and might as well get all their investigations done at once. Therefore, some sleep clinics mandate a full night in the sleep laboratory for almost all their patients as a standard feature of diagnosis and treatment.

Today, in large part because much has been published about sleep hygiene in the last 15 years, most insomnia patients know of and have tried a few if not all sleep-hygiene measures before coming to a sleep clinic. Although every clinic has slightly different diagnostic and treatment procedures, almost any one will advise the patient to undertake a sleep-hygiene program before going to the considerable expense of spending a night in the sleep laboratory.

Post-surgical laboratory measurement of sleep apnea poses even more profound problems than the measurement of insomnia. Treatment for sleep apnea is often surgical. In most cases, laboratory measurements reveal the condition and the laboratory monitoring helps ensure that surgery will help the patient. Many sleep-apnea patients report feeling hugely better after surgical revision of the upper airway (see chap. 10), and the patients' families and colleagues confirm improvements. But the sleep-laboratory measurements show improvement in only some of the patients—about half on average. This conflict has made many doctors wary of upper airway revision in treatment of sleep apnea.

The patients' subjective reports may be due to the placebo response, a worrisome consideration. Still, the placebo response in these cases is not very likely. Although the placebo response may be strong in treating insomnia—wakefulness—placebos generally do not work for excessive sleepiness, which is a primary characteristic of sleep apnea.

In addition, a strong case can be made that post-surgical laboratory monitoring may not reflect how the patients lived before surgery. As one doctor at Brigham and Women's Hospital Sleep Clinic in Boston discovered, some patients attending their post-operative laboratory session had discontinued caffeine, gained weight, resumed drinking, gotten little sleep the night before, or were more sensitive to the laboratory hardware attached to them, any of which affected how well they slept both at home and at the lab and how sleepy or alert they were at the lab. Both the average pre- and postoperative measurements and the variations from the average fluctuated widely. In other words, the doctor found he could not rely on the averages; biological improvements made by surgery were lost in the complexity of the patients' lives. It was more important to believe the patients' and patients' families' reports than to rely on lab results. (But laboratory monitoring can detect a decrease in blood-oxygen levels during sleep—a condition sometimes worth treating no matter how the patient feels.)

Despite difficulties objectively measuring the extent of the problem and analyzing the results, patients at a sleep clinic have one great advantage over many other patients undergoing medical treatment. They have a clearly defined goal—better sleep—and can tell promptly whether or not a given treatment is working. Where some ailments are concerned, a patient may have to wait weeks or even months to see if a given treatment has desirable effects. The patient at a sleep clinic, however, receives immediate feedback from how he or she sleeps. If you feel alert after sleep therapy, the treatment worked. If you still feel poorly, it failed. And if it failed, some other approach is indicated.

13
....

Sleeping Pills

Pills intended to induce sleep are among the most widely prescribed drugs in the United States. Sleeping pills can help relieve the temporary insomnia due to a sudden change in schedule or pain from an injury, for example. But when used over a long period of time, the pills tend to lose their effectiveness. Furthermore, sleeping pills can be habit-forming and can worsen sleep quality. The pills may also cause unpleasant side effects including hangover, energy loss, memory problems, and impaired coordination. Some people claim that only their nightly sleeping pill stands between them and insomnia, but in reality their pills are probably masking drug-withdrawal insomnia, not the original insomnia—the cause of which disappeared long ago.

Sleeping pills go by many names because drugs are divided into different categories, which include chemical structure, profile of physiological actions, or clinical use. Thus there is no essential difference between a sedative, a minor tranquilizer, and a sleeping pill, which is also known as a hypnotic. They all depress alertness. (Major tranquilizers do not sedate so much as relieve symptoms of psychosis.)

Statistics on the use of sleeping pills are impressive. An estimated 15 million Americans take prescription medications to induce sleep. Older people are the heaviest users of sleeping pills; roughly 50 percent of women and 25 percent of men over age 65 occasionally use some type of sedative to help them sleep. Overall, about 2 percent of American men and 3 percent of American women use prescription sleeping pills. Another 3 percent of the population relies on over-the-counter, nonprescription compounds—not counting alcoholic beverages—to help bring on sleep.

The occasional sleeping pill will not draw the user inevitably into the throes of drug dependency, any more than an occasional glass of wine with dinner will turn the drinker into an alcoholic. Sparing, intermittent use of hypnotics to achieve sleep usually poses no great danger. But long-term use of drugs to bring on sleep can lead to physiological drug dependency. At the same time, sleeping-pill use may merely mask the underlying cause of sleeplessness, which remains undetected. Thus the pill taker ends up with two problems—drug habituation and a sleep disorder—where previously he or she had only one.

OTHER EFFECTS OF SLEEPING PILLS

Thousands of people with chronic insomnia have found that pills do not bring them the sound sleep they were hoping for. Sleep induced by pills may be poor in quality, as researchers discovered when they monitored the sleep of individuals who took sleeping pills before going to bed. The EEGs of these sleepers were markedly different from those of people who enjoyed normal, undrugged slumber. But the more relevant comparison is not between drugged insomnia patients and normal sleepers but between drugged and undrugged poor sleepers.

A 1974 study by Dr. Anthony Kales and his colleagues at the Hershey Medical Center monitored the sleep of insomnia patients taking pentobarbital and other hypnotic drugs, and the sleep of a control group of insomnia patients receiving no sleeping pills, through the various stages of sleep from wakefulness to stage 4. Each group was observed over eight-hour periods at night, and the control group of drug-free insomnia patients actually slept more soundly overall than the sleeping-pill users did.

The insomniacs who took sleeping pills awoke almost twice as often during the night as the control group did and showed no deep sleep (stages 3 and 4) whatsoever. By contrast, the typical insomniac in the control group managed 30 to 45 minutes of deep sleep. The amount of REM sleep also was less in the drug-using group. A chart of these results made strikingly clear the instability of drug-induced sleep: whereas sleepers in the control group were typically able to sleep for perhaps 45 minutes at a stretch before returning briefly to wakefulness, the pill users' charts indicated they had been able to sleep only 15 minutes or so at a time on average (see fig. 11).

Abnormality of the EEG is even more pronounced in persons who have abruptly withdrawn from sleeping-pill use. Deprived of the drug, the electrical activity in the drug-habituated brain changes significantly. REM sleep especially increases and the sleeper is liable to have nightmares, although this becomes less likely when withdrawal from the drug is gradual. There is drug hangover—a sluggish, groggy feeling in the morning much like that experienced after heavy drinking. Even the performance of tasks done the following afternoon may be affected.

Some drugs are metabolized into longer-acting substances. For example, diazepam (Valium) is turned into the metabolite desmethyldiazepam; a methyl group, or basic molecular fragment with one carbon atom, is removed from the diazepam molecule. Similarly, an alkyl group, or molecule fragment with a chain of carbon atoms, is removed from flurazepam (Dalmane) to make desalkylflurazepam. The body metabolizes these substances slowly. It takes a long time—about 100 hours on average, with wide variations among individuals—for the blood levels of desmethyldiazepam and desalkylflurazepam to decrease by a half. During this 100 hours, and well beyond it, the drug still acts on the nervous system. Depending on the person, some of this action may be therapeutic. For instance, the person may have an easier time falling asleep one, two, or even three nights after taking the medication, or he or she may feel less anxious (another symptom diazepam alleviates) the following day. Also,

Hours after bedtime are shown on the horizontal axis, sleep stages on the vertical axis. Light areas indicate REM sleep. Notice that the control patient takes one hour to fall asleep and that the patient awakens more than one hour prior to arising. The drug-taking patient also takes almost an hour to fall asleep and, in addition, experiences no deep sleep and more frequent wakeful periods. REM sleep is decreased as well. The long wakeful period at the end of the night, however, has been broken up.

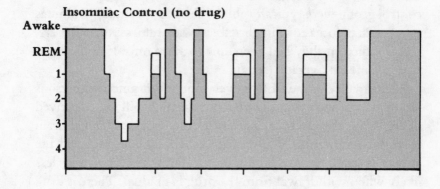

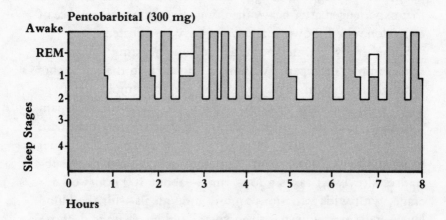

Figure 11 Sleeping patterns of a patient who chronically used pentobarbital compared to a composite of insomnia patients not taking medication.

the person may have fewer drug-withdrawal symptoms when he or she discontinues a slowly excreted drug, because the gradual diminution of drug levels prevents the precipitous drops that bring on sudden withdrawal symptoms.

On the other hand, the long-acting effects may be therapeutic but they may also produce unwanted side effects, such as hangover or a lack of coordination. What might be welcome tranquilization for an anxious young person, who has a higher metabolic rate of the nervous system, greater alertness, and more capacity to deal with sedatives, can turn into grogginess or incompetence in the older person who has some infirmities.

The above are generalizations. There are young people who have terrible hangovers from even short-acting medications and older people who occasionally use long-acting medications with some benefits; for instance, an 81-year-old woman who finds relief from restless legs syndrome through use of diazepam.

SLEEPING PILLS AND THE PLACEBO EFFECT

Just as with prescription sleeping pills, over-the-counter sleeping compounds sell briskly. But as a rule, these drugs contain so weak a sedative that their direct effects are slight. When they seem to work at all, they owe much of their efficacy to the placebo effect; they appear to work, but mostly because the user expects them to. Most of these pills contain diphenhydramine (Benadryl) or doxylomine (Unisom), which are antihistamines with sedative actions.

The placebo effect's power to induce sleep demonstrates faith in medicine. The user is prepared psychologically for sleep, but needs the extra psychological "boost" supplied by the pill, even though the pill in itself is virtually without any physical effects. To find out whether an over-the-counter pill works or not, researchers have collected information from hospital inpatients about their sleep after they have taken such pills, and compared this with statements by patients after they took placebo pills. Additional research has compared the effect of over-the-counter medications and placebo pills on the sleep of insomnia patients.

The general impression arising from such studies is that over-the-counter medications do not relieve insomnia any more than placebo pills, although some may have a hypnotic effect. Nevertheless, the placebo effect can really help.

One over-the-counter pill not marketed for insomnia, but possibly helpful for it, is aspirin. A study by Drs. Peter Hauri and Peter Silberfarb at Dartmouth found that aspirin improved the sleep of insomnia patients who were monitored in the sleep laboratory. Aspirin-taking subjects slept significantly better than those taking placebos. The study also found that aspirin's action apparently did not depend on its pain-relieving effect, and that some insomnia patients were helped more than others. In fact, aspirin's profile as a hypnotic drug could be compared with several prescription hypnotics. In clinical experience, older people seem to be the ones who use aspirin to relieve their insomnia.

Nonetheless, about 3 percent of all adults in the United States find over-the-counter sleeping aids so effective that they buy them on occasion. If these people were only buying simple sugar pills for their placebo effect, the pills probably would be perfectly safe. But some ingredients in these over-the-counter pills may have significant side effects that include nervousness, loss of memory, and unsteadiness. So over-the-counter sleeping pills are not wholly harmless, and purchasers should be aware of both their limited utility and their possible side effects.

The placebo effect also applies to prescription sleeping pills. Not all their action is attributable to chemical action. Much depends also on the patient's faith in the drug's power. One interesting study conducted in Milan, Italy, compared the sleep-inducing effect of a placebo pill with that of 100 milligrams of phenobarbital in a group of 78 middle-age patients. The patients were not told which kind of pill they were taking, nor were the nurses who distributed the pills so informed. The morning after taking the pills, patients with mild insomnia who received the placebo reported they had slept just as well as patients who had received phenobarbital. It appears the placebo effect went only so far, however, because patients with severe insomnia reported far better results from the phenobarbital.

RISKS ASSOCIATED WITH SLEEPING PILLS

The importance of the placebo effect should not be allowed to overshadow the fact that sleeping pills are strong medicine and should be given some healthy respect. Under some circumstances, the use of sleeping pills carries considerable risk. For one thing, they may interact with other drugs. For example, alcohol enhances the effect of other sedatives. It may add to or else multiply the effect of a sedative, or prolong its action. The exact nature of this interaction will depend on how tolerant and sensitive the individual is to the alcohol and the other drug taken together, to the dose of both drugs, and to how the drug effects are measured.

A small amount of alcohol that might not cause impairment on its own may have its effects increased suddenly when taken in combination with sleeping pills. The pill taker who also drinks may find that alcohol suddenly affects him or her much more. Alcohol not only increases the sedative effect of sleeping pills, but also may slow down the excretion of the medication from the body, thus prolonging its effect. As we will see in a moment, taking sleeping pills with alcohol just before bedtime is especially dangerous for some people, because it invites impaired breathing.

The actions of many other prescription drugs can also be modified by sleeping pills. Some prescription drugs, for example anticonvulsants, antidepressants, and antihypertensive medications, have sedative actions of their own. Other drugs without sedative actions may also be affected. The sedative chloral hydrate accelerates the metabolism of some blood-thinning medications like dicumarol or warfarin (Coumadin), which are prescribed for vascular disease. So a person taking warfarin who also begins taking chloral hydrate may develop slightly thickened blood and will need to have the dose of blood thinner raised.

Of course, the prescribing doctor should try to prevent such problems. But this can be difficult for several reasons.

First, there are so many over-the-counter and prescribed drugs that no one can keep track of all their possible interactions.

Second, many people's medical care these days is divided among several doctors, with no one doctor in charge. It is hard for any one of those doctors to know all the drugs a patient may be taking. Sometimes, but not always, a pharmacist will call doctors to see if they are aware of all the pills a patient is taking. But it is primarily the doctor's responsibility to know if the patient is already taking other drugs that could interact with the one prescribed. (Patients may patronize several drugstores, making it still more difficult for doctors and druggists to keep track of their medication.)

Third, many people take such a large number of medications that they cannot remember them all, or they may forget to bring a complete list for the doctor's review. And it may happen that a patient must take two drugs even when an interaction between them is recognized.

Finally, some patients who want a drug will not take no for an answer. They will shop around until they find a doctor who will honor their request for a prescription.

Therefore, so many people are taking so many different kinds of medication that drug interactions are common. On admission to a hospital, many people, especially people over 65, are discovered to be taking 5 to 10 types of pills daily. This "polypharmacy" approach to modern medicine is illustrated by an anecdote about the famous cardiologist Samuel Levine.

Making the rounds one day with interns and residents at a Boston hospital, Dr. Levine was told that one patient was on 14 medications.

"Stop all but two," Levine said.

"Which two?" asked a resident.

"Any two," Levine replied.

Dr. Levine's remark hyperbolically arraigned polypharmacy. Undoubtedly he meant to caution the doctors about the gravity of multiple drug prescriptions. His suggestion sounds realistic, however, for the many patients with multiple medical problems who are treated with an array of laxatives, analgesics, hypnotics, diuretics, tranquilizers, eye drops, antidepressants, and antiarrhythmic and antibronchospastic drugs.

Accidental or deliberate overdose is another risk of sleeping pills. In most cases, a sleeping-pill overdose kills by inhibiting respiration. Large amounts of sleeping-pill medication can impair function of the lower-brain centers that govern breathing and other vital body functions. Normal coughing as well as the gag reflex, which prevents food and liquids from going down the windpipe, also may be prevented by a sleeping-pill overdose. The normal tendency to swallow saliva and lung secretions as well as regurgitated stomach juices may be impaired too. These secretions may therefore enter the bronchial airways, causing inflammation or endangering breathing.

The danger of suicidal overdose from sleeping pills is especially great for insomnia patients, many of whom also suffer from depression. With this hazard in mind, when a sleeping pill is thought advisable, doctors have taken to prescribing benzodiazepine drugs such as Valium, with which it is very hard to kill yourself. To consume a dangerous dose of Valium, about 2,500 milligrams, you would have to swallow 500 pills, an undertaking involving considerable time and effort, not to mention huge amounts of water.

On the other hand, a person can easily take a dangerous overdose of sleeping pills by accident if he or she washes them down with alcohol. A drink will magnify the effects of sleeping pills and make an inadvertent, fatal overdose that much more likely.

In 1985 an article by Dr. Charles Reynolds and his colleagues from the Sleep Evaluation Center at the Western Psychiatric Center in Pittsburgh appeared with the title "Sleeping Pills for the Elderly: Are They Ever Justified?" Those over 65 represent about 15 percent of the population, but consume more than a third of the sleeping pills prescribed, which in itself raises questions about whether such disproportionate use is justified. The mere fact that Reynolds's question could be open to discussion at all suggests that many sleeping pills are used irresponsibly. The article concluded with the usual plea for minimal, intermittent, and monitored use of sleeping pills and use of other measures to foster good sleep.

Why then are sleeping pills prescribed at all, if their use is so questionable? The answer: Sleeping pills do work well, but only under limited conditions. They do promote sleep in people who use them only rarely. Such people are in the majority: People who use sleeping pills fewer than 30 times a year account for most sleeping-pill use. What is not helpful (and possibly harmful) is long-term use to remedy chronic insomnia. Where chronic insomnia is concerned, sleeping pills may purchase temporary relief for the user, but at a long-term cost paid by side effects, harmful drug interactions, ineffectiveness, and withdrawal symptoms.

14
....

Psychotherapy

Psychotherapy can help relieve the anxiety that worsens sleep. It does not change a troublesome situation in life, but it helps you cope with it by relieving inner conflicts. A person who thinks psychotherapy might improve his or her sleep may wish to consult a specialist. But desirable results are not guaranteed, and the treatment is both time-consuming and expensive.

Most psychotherapy is undertaken in hopes of alleviating much vaguer symptoms than insomnia or disturbed-sleep problems. Relating poorly with other people or feeling that something is missing in life or being depressed or having anxiety, which itself is a symptom of a host of problems, bring many people to the psychotherapist's office. No systematic studies have explored whether psychotherapy helps insomnia, and even if the outcome of such research showed that psychotherapy worsened insomnia, the interpretation of such a result would remain controversial. Some would say that insomnia is not relieved by psychotherapy, but others might propose that therapy was still useful because it uncovered previously unconscious feelings that allowed the person to try to deal with them directly. Even if the patient's sleep worsened, it might be suggested that other repressed feelings—a health problem, a behavioral blowup—might have afflicted the insomnia patient in the future.

If a patient decides to embark on a psychotherapy program aimed at improving sleep, at least he or she has a defined goal. It might be worthwhile for the patient to estimate approximately how long it will take before he or she judges whether the sleep problem is or is not relieved. Later on this will prevent the patient from indecisively languishing in a psychotherapy program.

ANXIETY AND INSOMNIA

The aim of psychotherapy is to reduce the anxiety that results when a person's wishes conflict with the requirements of society or when a person is torn between conflicting wishes.

If a family member or a colleague at work fights with or berates a person, the age-old fight-or-flight response, inherited from the distant past, might urge the person either to attack the other party or to turn and flee. Neither of those options is acceptable from a social standpoint, however, so the person must choose some other more tactful but less instinct-bound way of handling the situation. The person might decide to do and say nothing—just sit and wait for the attacker to finish and go away. This is a socialized, nonviolent solution to the disagreement, but at the cost of strong tension between society's strictures and ancient instincts. Such tension creates anxiety, which in turn can interfere with sleep. If this sleep-robbing anxiety existed purely on the conscious level, where it was directly perceived, coping with it would be a straightforward process. But anxiety also lies much deeper.

There is an unconscious level of anxiety that reaches deep into the mind, like the roots of a tree. Dealing with this less accessible unconscious anxiety is difficult, because the conscious mind does the dealing. Yet this deep-seated anxiety must be addressed somehow if it generates a sleep disorder; in some cases, psychotherapy may confront the problem at its source.

Perhaps anxiety does not directly explain insomnia. Rather,

anxiety and insomnia might both grow out of an overdeveloped tendency toward alertness (see chap. 6). But anxious people may find it harder to stay organized enough or to control themselves enough to keep sleep charts, discontinue use of drugs, or exercise regularly—all the things needed to encourage good sleep. For anxious people, many of the treatments for sleep apnea—for example, C-PAP, surgery, weight loss, and discontinuation of sedatives—are much harder to cope with. Thus lessening the anxiety—or feelings of resentment about needing such treatment—might free a person to carry out other sleep treatments.

PSYCHOTHERAPY AS A TREATMENT FOR INSOMNIA

Many people assume that psychotherapy is the best way to relieve insomnia. When they telephone sleep clinics, they presume that they will be seen regularly to discuss their feelings and that this procedure will relieve them. Yet, as discussed, much serious insomnia and sleepiness are due to causes that are not remedied by psychotherapy, such as drug sensitivities or scheduling problems.

Psychotherapy can help greatly, however, in one particular situation: when the patient does not follow the measures that are likely to relieve his or her sleep problem. Changing entrenched habits requires determination. To quit smoking or to get up at a regular early arising time is not easy for many people, even when they know they should do so. For psychotherapy to be effective, the individual must feel a conflict over his or her own behavior, must wish to change it, and must have some willingness to transform his or her wishes into action. Psychotherapy alone is seldom the complete answer to sleep disorders aggravated by anxiety. But the therapist can hope to eliminate some troublesome ways of thinking that have trapped a patient into poor sleep habits.

One might say that many insomnia patients are prisoners of their own behavior, and that psychotherapy helps release them, even if therapy is not the key itself.

SLEEP DISTURBANCE RELIEVED
BY PSYCHOTHERAPY

Ms. K. consulted a sleep clinic seeking help for insomnia. The first consultation revealed that she was full of anger. Her bottled-up rage had been accumulating since childhood, when she had to cope with a violent, alcoholic stepfather. In high school, she spent much of her time studying and generally avoided other students.

After graduation, she worked as a flight attendant for a major airline. A tall, attractive woman, she suddenly found herself the focus of attention from some interesting and successful men. Yet she felt uncomfortable when they showed such interest, and she never allowed any of these relationships to develop beyond a certain point—until she met one very handsome, wealthy, sophisticated man and married him.

The marriage disappointed her. She had expected her new husband to stay home much of the time so they could enjoy each other. Instead, he spent much of his time away from home, frequenting bars. He also told her that he had no interest in having children, whereas she wanted very much to have a family. Ms. K. found herself trapped in an unsatisfactory marriage and received little emotional support from anyone. In addition, she had to contend with unwanted sexual overtures from a male neighbor.

In short, all of Ms. K.'s experiences with men perpetuated a fear that men were predators and would victimize her if given the opportunity. Lonely and downhearted, she would lie awake in bed long after retiring, musing angrily on how life had mistreated her. At last she would fall asleep, only to be tormented by threatening dreams. The next morning, she would awaken edgy and irritable.

She tried to cope with her restless sleep as she had done with all other aspects of her life, by following a rigid, complex routine. She would start preparing for bedtime 90 minutes in advance, starting with an elaborate bathtime ritual. Next she would inspect everything in the bedroom to make sure all was as it should be, windowshades in the right position and bedclothes arranged perfectly. She even observed a complex ritual of rolling first to one side and then the other, to let her heart, as she explained it, come to rest on the left side of her chest.

Symptoms of anxiety often symbolize unconscious thoughts. Rituals like Ms. K.'s might mean "If I make everything correct, my problems will be solved." The underlying meaning of the ritual rolling from side to side might be interpreted as "I have to get my heart in the right place." The meanings of such symptoms emerge as the patient feels free to discuss conflicts and topics about which she was ashamed.

Treating Ms. K.'s sleep problem was difficult, partly because it was difficult for her to trust her psychiatrist, who was male. Her long-standing, pent-up anger toward men had to be overcome.

Over the next three and a half years, Ms. K. and her psychiatrist proceeded one step at a time. Together they established that she was angry at him, first as a male physician and second for trying to make her give up some of the habits that were interfering with her sleep. For example, her elaborate prebedtime rituals made her bedroom a place of intense activity rather than rest. Also, Ms. K. resisted her psychiatrist's efforts to help because, once again, she was afraid that she was putting a man in a position to victimize her.

Eventually, Ms. K. understood that through her bedtime rituals she compensated for a deep-rooted sense of shame and failure. They granted her only a momentary illusion of perfection.

Even so, years passed before Ms. K. made her first serious effort to rid herself of sleep-robbing habits. At last she relented, started keeping a sleep chart, and gave up coffee. She also took up progressive relaxation exercises to relieve hyperarousal insomnia. The exercises actually increased her anxiety at first, because they resembled the pre-bedtime rituals that for years had been keeping her from refreshing sleep.

But eventually these techniques, together with a self-understanding she gained from psychotherapy, helped improve Ms. K.'s sleep and, moreover, her life as a whole. Her nights of troubled sleep grew less and less frequent. She even had the confidence to talk to her husband about her dissatisfaction, and he invested more of himself in the marriage.

A QUESTION OF PRIORITIES

The question of whether Ms. K. truly benefited from psychotherapy is controversial. Was relief from insomnia really the greatest benefit of the therapy? After all, Ms. K. still felt some loneliness and still had no children. But consider the psychotherapy contract. Her loneliness and desire for children were not at issue in her treatment. What she wanted was help sleeping, and that was what she got.

Some psychiatrists might say Ms. K.'s therapist neglected more important problems or worsened them, to the extent that her sleeplessness was related to them, and that without insomnia she would be less interested in them and/or less motivated to work on them. Some might also argue that he colluded with her to ignore important areas of her life.

This is a matter of values and opinions, on which both professionals and laypersons hold different beliefs. Her doctor did not believe he could order Ms. K.'s priorities for her or suggest what she ought to do, as opposed to what she wished to do. Still, some would say that since Ms. K. was seeking help, she should have had the benefit of a close observer's recommendation for working on her other problems as well, even if she did not articulate those problems plainly. There is no clear and easy resolution to such a controversy, which probably will persist as long as psychotherapy is practiced.

As Ms. K.'s history shows, psychotherapy used in combination with other therapies, such as relaxation exercises, may help relieve sleep problems.

COULD YOU BENEFIT
FROM PSYCHOTHERAPY?

If you have insomnia, chances are you do not need psychotherapy to relieve it. You are much more likely to improve your
sleep using other, less expensive, and less time-consuming
methods, such as practicing the sleep-hygiene program described in chapter 11. After establishing good sleep hygiene,
more specific causes of the insomnia can be diagnosed and
treated, such as disorders of the biological clocks or depression.

If you cannot do what is necessary to improve your sleep,
such as giving up nicotine or other sleep-affecting drugs, then
psychotherapy may help. In any event, if insomnia is giving
you serious difficulty, and you cannot take basic steps to overcome it, discussing the possible usefulness of psychotherapy
with your doctor cannot harm you and may open a productive
avenue for dealing with your sleep problem.

Index

213